DOCTOR SEBI DIET

The Ultimate Cookbook to Lose Weight and Enhance Your Body's Performances thanks to Dr Sebi TRUE Teachings and Herbs. Including 101 plant-based, Alkaline, and Electric Recipes

By Dorothy Vandekamp

© **Copyright 2020 by Dorothy Vandekamp - All rights reserved.**

The content contained within this book may not be reproduced, duplicated, or transmitted without direct written permission from the author or the publisher.

Under no circumstances will any blame or legal responsibility be held against the publisher, or author, for any damages, reparation, or monetary loss due to the information contained within this book. Either directly or indirectly.

Legal Notice:

This book is copyright protected. This book is only for personal use. You cannot amend, distribute, sell, use, quote, or paraphrase any part, or the content within this book, without the consent of the author or publisher.

Disclaimer Notice:

Please note the information contained within this document is for educational and entertainment purposes only. All effort has been executed to present accurate, up-to-date, and reliable, complete information.

No warranties of any kind are declared or implied. Readers acknowledge that the author is not engaging in the rendering of legal, financial, medical, or professional advice. The content within this book has been derived from various sources. Please consult a licensed professional before attempting any techniques outlined in this book.

By reading this document, the reader agrees that under no circumstances is the author responsible for any losses, direct or indirect, which are incurred as a result of the use of the information contained within this document, including, but not limited to, — errors, omissions, or inaccuracies.

TABLE OF CONTENTS

INTRODUCTION 8

CHAPTER 1: WHAT IS THE EXACT RECOMMENDED DIET FROM DR SEBI? 10

Who was the Doctor Sebi? 10

Where did he Learn his Healing Knowledge? 10

    Sues Dr. Sebi in New York Supreme Court 11

    The philosophy of Dr. Sebi 12

How is Mucus Removed? 12

    What were Dr. Sebi's favorite foods? 12

    Is Doctor Sebi's diet healthy and safe? 13

8 Important Rules to Perfectly Follow the Dr. Sebi Diet 14

The cons of the Dr. Sebi diet 15

CHAPTER 2: DOCTOR SEBI'S PROCEDURE TO EFFECTIVELY LOSE WEIGHT 18

Dr. Sebi Food List 19

    Vegetables: 19

    Fruits: 20

    Nuts and seeds: 21

    Spices – seasonings: 21

    Sugars: 21

    All-natural herbal teas: 22

    Oils: 22

Foods to Avoid 23

CHAPTER 3: DOCTOR SEBI DIET'S BENEFITS 25

Dr. Sebi Diet's 7-Day Meal Plan (Alkaline Diet Plan) 25

Frequently Asked Questions 27

CHAPTER 4: BREAKFAST RECIPES 30

1. Spelled bread without yeast.. 30
2. Puff pastry - quiche with broccoli and camembert.. 31
3. Muesli basic mix 32
4. Spelled bread with sunflower seeds 33
5. Fruit buckwheat porridge with pomegranate seeds 34
6. Buckwheat semolina 35
7. Maroni coconut cream "Symphony of the trees" 36
8. Dark chocolate cream with figs... 36
9. Apple and coconut cream 37
10. Apple and almond muesli mandarins.. 38
11. Danny's morning hour - basic breakfast buffet... 39
12. Basic breakfast buffet with buckwheat 40
13. Basic cereal 41
14. Fruit salad with strawberries and tigernuts 42
15. Oatmeal Seasoned with Vegetables 42
16. Blackberry and lemon muffins for tea 44
17. Cherry and poppy seed muffins.. 45
18. Cocoa, banana, and whole-grain spelled flour muffins.. 46

CHAPTER 5: SNACK RECIPES 48

19. Homemade granola 48
20. Low carb poppy seed cake... 49
21. Refreshing Blueberry Bites with Nutri-Plus Lemon Cake 50
22. Chia Protein Energy Balls 50
23. Protein bars for the extra portion of the power... 51
24. Delicious Cinnamon Stars with Nutri-Plus Hazelnut 52
25. Low carb poppy seed cake... 53
26. Refreshing Blueberry Bites with Nutri-Plus Lemon Cake 54
27. Chia Protein Energy Balls 54

28.	Protein bars for the extra portion of the power	55
29.	Mango Nice Cream	56
30.	Sweet hummus dip for snacking	56
31.	Energy balls made from chickpeas	57
32.	The healthy fruit bread for snacking	58
33.	Creamy protein chocolate with quinoa	60

CHAPTER 6: VEGETABLE RECIPES 63

34.	Boar Stew with Vegetables, Herbs and Plums, Tuscan Recipe	63
35.	Turkish Acma With Sheep's Cheese and Vegetables	64
36.	My creamy, vegan peanut fritters with vegetables and soy	65
37.	Bolognese Sauce with Lots of Vegetables	67
38.	Vegetables - Lasagna A La Mousse	68
39.	Fried Noodles with Vegetables and Meat (Asian)	69
40.	Salmon with Vegetables and Potatoes	70
41.	Fried Salmon on Mediterranean Vegetables	72
42.	Oven Chicken with Vegetables	74
43.	Beef Steak with Mustard and Herb Topping and Vegetables	76
44.	Protein Cream Biscuits	76
45.	Protein Cream Biscuits Chocolate Cookies From A Few Ingredients	77
46.	Vegan Protein Pancakes Fluffy Pancakes Without Eggs	78
47.	Vegan Brownies Recipe Juicy, Chocolaty, Sugar-Free	79
48.	Protein Chia Pudding with Irresistible Chocolate Candy	79
49.	Oatmeal Seasoned with Vegetables	80
50.	Crushed Olives Paste	81

CHAPTER 7: SMOOTHIES AND JUICES 83

51.	Carrot Drink with Parsley and Lemon with Garlic	83
52.	Spicy tomato-thick milk drink	83
53.	Apple Cherry Cocktail with Celery	84
54.	Apple Vegetable Juice with Beetroot	84

55.	Strong vegetable juice with ginger	85
56.	Fast Beetroot Drink with Chives	85
57.	Paprika Cocktail with orange	86
58.	Red Apple Juice with Red Cabbage	86
59.	Spicy Carrot Juice with Curry Foam	86
60.	Cucumber-orange drink	87
61.	Cucumber drink with wasabi	87
62.	Cucumber Smoothie	88
63.	Cucumber smoothie with muesli	88
64.	Cucumber and Blackberry Smoothie	89
65.	Spicy carrot drink	90
66.	Green Smoothies with Yogurt	90

CHAPTER 8: DESSERT RECIPES 93

67.	Healthy Samoa's Smoothie	93
68.	Healthy raspberry thumbprint cookies	95
69.	Healthy blueberry lemon ricotta parfaits	97
70.	Healthy chocolate chip cookies	97
71.	Healthy key lime pie dip	99
72.	Healthy oatmeal raisin cookies	99
73.	Healthy Black Velvet Chia Seed Pudding	101
74.	Healthy Cake Batter Milkshake	102
75.	Healthy Pumpkin Ice Cream	103
76.	Baked oatmeal à la Pumpkin Pie	104
77.	Pumpkin spiced macarons	105
78.	Homemade Chocolate Chip Cookies Recipe	107
79.	Pumpkin swirl brownies	108
80.	Chocolate peanut squares	109
81.	Nougat Whims	110
82.	Cheesecake mousse with raspberries	111

CHAPTER 9: SALAD RECIPES 114

83.	Chickpea salad	114
84.	Salad with Avocado, Pineapple and Cucumbers	115
85.	Mango with avocado salad	116
86.	Avocado and lettuce salad	117
87.	Vegan Vegetable Mini Tortillas	118
88.	Broccoli Soup, Green Leaves, And Beans	119
89.	Baked omelet with baby spinach	120
90.	Vegetarian recipe	121
91.	Raw Vegetables. Chopped Salad	122
92.	Mediterranean Veggie Pita Sandwich	124
93.	Classic asparagus	125
94.	Soup cream from palm heart	126
95.	Broccoli Soup, Green Leaves, And Beans	127

CHAPTER 10: SOUP AND STEW RECIPES 130

96.	Nopal Soup	130
97.	Vegetable broth without sodium	130
98.	Comforting noodle and chickpea soup	131
99.	Soup loaded with miso noodles	132
100.	"Bone" mineral broth and vegetables	133
101.	Noodle soup with broccoli and ginger	134

CONCLUSION 137

Where does Dr. Sebi believe disease come from? 137

INTRODUCTION

Dr. Sebi's diet is a dietary approach not approved by mainstream medicine, which essentially relies on a mucus-free diet (like Arnold Ehret's mucus-free diet). Dr Sebi (real name Alfredo Bowman, who passed away in 2016) in the 1980s aroused great interest internationally because his diet was considered to cure many diseases of the modern era.

At the moment, however, on Dr. Sebi's website, it is written that the diet does not replace the doctor's opinion and is not designed to cure illnesses but to detoxify.

Dr. Sebi's diet includes some types of vegetables, almost all fruit except hybrid varieties, seeds, nuts, butter from seeds or nuts, vegetable oils, teas, herbs, spices, and some whole grains. Legumes (apart from some), meat, fish, eggs, and dairy products are excluded. We can say that Dr. Sebi's diet is therefore a vegan diet with some restrictions.

In this eBook, we will explain everything you need to know about Dr. Sebi's diet, the benefit of it, and more.

CHAPTER 1: WHAT IS THE EXACT RECOMMENDED DIET FROM DR SEBI?

Who was the Doctor Sebi?

In this book, we will talk about the great Dr. Sebi. His beginnings, how he started in the world of healing, his relapses, and his philosophy.

A guy ahead of his time and with a great humanitarian interest, honest and with great pride. Now we will give a brief review of its history and later of its philosophy.

Alfredo Bowman was an herbalist, born on November 26, 1933, in La Ceiba, Honduras. Then he settled in the United States, where his work became more recognized. He passed away on August 6, 2016, at the age of 82.

Better known as Dr. Sebi, he gained much notoriety for proclaiming the cure of different diseases, such as diabetes, HIV, herpes, lupus, among other ills. Also, he treated many celebrities, such as Michael Jackson and Lisa "Left Eye" Lopes of the musical group TLC.

With a totally naturist style, he believed that any disease could be cured through food and fasting, which for the time, was unthinkable. It still is. He acquired his knowledge in a self-taught way, so he was not a doctor recognized by the medical community.

It all started, after having treated his diabetes without success, he immigrated to Mexico, where he met a local herbalist, by the name of Alfredo Cortez. In that place, he found a cure for his disease, accompanied by obesity, impotence, and asthma. After being cured of these ills, he decided to dedicate himself fully to health.

Where did he Learn his Healing Knowledge?

He dedicated his life to the study of herbs from North, South, and Central America and Africa, and the Caribbean. Learned much next to his grandmother "Mama Hay" of Haitian descent, with whom he shared time learning about nature and plants. Years later, Dr. Sebi who moved to the United States was diagnosed with diabetes, overweight, asthma, and even impotence. After unsuccessful attempts to be treated by conventional doctors, he recommended that he seek treatment in Cuernavaca with a Mexican herbalist, Alfredo Cortez.

Who explained to him that his illnesses were the product of his poor diet, the Mexican recommended him to fast for 90 days but Sebi fasted for 94. "Did you do it?" Cortez asked him, when Sebi returned to Mexico from Los Angeles, California, to which Sebi replied, "Yes ... I feel relaxed and calm for the first time in my life." Cortez explained, "Good, what was happening with you was that you were disobeying the black culture and tradition.

It means that black people live by a law that does not come from philosophy, it is a law that comes directly from the nature of the deepest part of life, the understanding of life. "Dr. Sebi was always grateful to the herbalist and God for being cured. " A Mexican cured me and I want to learn more about these plants." From that day on, Dr. Sebi dedicated himself to creating compounds for cleansing and revitalizing the body's cells. In 1987 he was arrested in New York, facing charges for practicing medicine without a license and for selling non-FDA approved products and for claiming to cure cancer, AIDS.

Dr. Sebi asked the State three key questions, being his defense,

"True or not true that the bible teaches us that ... plants are for medicine?"

"Second question, is it true or not true that Mr. Hippocrates, the father gave me medicine that cured all diseases ... did he use chemicals or plants?"

"True or not true that the human body is carbon-based? ... the substance that complements a carbon-based body must also be carbon-based ... Chemical affinity. There is compatibility ... conduction."

And with these questions, Dr. Sebi won the case, since his opponents could not fight with these answers. The Judge asked him how he had come to such an understanding. To which Dr. Sebi replied, "I don't know, but it started with a Mexican Mrs. Judge and the rest has to be God, and studying the plants ... "

For the rest of his life he dedicated himself to curing people, he opened the Usha Center (Usha Village) located in La Ceiba, Honduras, and has attended many celebrities such as Michael Jackson, Lisa Lopes, Steven Seagal, John Travolta, and Eddie Murphy. On May 28, 2016, Dr. Sebi was arrested at the Roatan, Honduras Airport, to declare the earnings he was bringing with his clinic in Los Angeles. He died on August 6, 2016.

Sues Dr. Sebi in New York Supreme Court

Proclaiming the cure of various "incurable" diseases led him to face charges for "practicing medicine without a license" in the Supreme Court of New York in 1988.

The most curious thing about this was that Dr. Sebi presented more than 70 patients with reliable proof that he had cured these diseases, a fact that made him win the trial and release him. This fact further triggered its popularity and acceptance among people.

The philosophy of Dr. Sebi

Dr. Sebi believed that all diseases could be cured through food, but above all, abstaining from the wrong foods. Following in the footsteps of the great Hippocrates, the father of medicine, he believed that using medicinal herbs, algae such as sea moss (or "sea moss") and consuming foods with a base pH, or alkaline, you could cure yourself of any illness.

Also, he was a faithful believer in fasting as a tool for healing. In fact, in his villa in Honduras, it was common for him to guide his patients by fasting for very long periods (40 days or more). In these fasts, they were only allowed to drink water, or make infusions, with different herbs or sea moss.

Another reason that Dr. Sebi became well known was because of his belief that there was only one reason that people got sick. His saying was, "There is only one cause of illness, and that is mucus. If you remove the mucus, you remove the disease.

How is Mucus Removed?

Mucus, according to Sebi, is eliminated by avoiding these 4 types of food: starch, meat, dairy, and sugar. For him, "blood and starch" were not food, that is, his diet did not include meat, dairy, eggs, rice, potatoes, pasta, among other foods. As you can see, his diet was very strict.

First, to starch he attributes problems to the liver, diseases such as cancer and tumors, because, according to his words, when it is digested, it produces carbonic acid, which would be responsible for causing the problems mentioned above.

As for meats, Sebi said they could cause ulcers in the digestive tract and stomach, and they also produce uric acid, which could lead to problems such as hypertension and heart attacks.

Dairy says that, like meat, they produce hypertension, increased cholesterol, and clogged arteries.

Finally, sugar, according to Sebi, would cause problems in the teeth, pancreas, kidneys, and brain. At the same time, it causes digestive issues. It produces neurotic behavior, the latter being very evident, especially in children, who tend to become very hyperactive when consuming a lot of sugar.

Dr. Sebi used to say that the body is electrical, so it needs food that is also electrical or "alive." This mainly includes fruits and vegetables.

And not only that, since many vegetables were also prohibited. He only allowed the foods that were "created by God" (in his words) to be the ones to be eaten. The above excludes foods such as broccoli, carrots, beans (or beans), cauliflower, or any food that is a hybrid of more species.

What were Dr. Sebi's favorite foods?

We are going to divide them by categories, with some examples of each case:

- **Grains:** Amaranth, barley, quinoa, or wild rice.
- **Nuts:** Walnuts, macadamias, sesame seeds, or hemp seeds.
- **Vegetables:** Cherry tomatoes, chickpeas, kale, avocados, cucumbers, mushrooms, onion, or pumpkin.
- **Fruits:** apples, bananas (only the small ones or "burritos"), berries, dates, seeded grapes, limes, mango, seeded melon, coconuts, soursop, papayas, or raisins with seeds.
- **Oils:** Coconut oil and olive oil (without heating), grape seed oil, sesame oil, or avocado oil.

To sweeten you can use date syrup or coconut sugar; to salt use sea salt, not table salt.

As you see, it is a pretty strict diet. These foods are the most accessible to most, which we have extracted from "Dr. Sebi approved" foods, as there are many others that are rare.

Also, Dr. Sebi placed great emphasis on iron intake. He said that it was impossible to get sick when the body was supplied with large amounts of iron. This mineral is essential for the blood, and it is the blood that provides the body and brain with oxygen, thus improving its functioning.

He also said that this is the only "magnetic" mineral, which causes more minerals to adhere to it, thus improving the supply of minerals we need on a day-to-day basis. Quite an interesting approach.

You may or may not agree with Dr. Sebi's beliefs, but that does not take away from the fact that he was a fascinating man, with a lot of wisdom and that he also left a legacy that will last for a long time. New trends point towards a more natural style, which this famous herbalist was an expert.

Perhaps in the future, we will have new practitioners of this discipline, with the willingness to improve people's quality of life.

Is Doctor Sebi's diet healthy and safe?

Dr. Sebi Diet is a herbal diet developed by the late Dr. It is said to rejuvenate your cells by removing toxic waste by alkalizing your blood.

The diet is based on a shortlist of approved foods and numerous supplements.

This chapter will review Dr. Sebi's diet's pros and cons and examine whether scientific evidence supports his health claims.

This diet is based on Dr. Sebi's African bio-mineral balance theory, developed by herbalist Alfredo Darrington Bowman-better. Despite his name, Dr. Sebi was not a doctor.

He designed this diet for anyone who naturally wants to cure or prevent disease and improve overall health without using conventional Western medicine.

According to Dr. Sebi, illness is the result of your body's mucus build-up. For example, lung mucus accumulation is pneumonia, while diabetes is an excess of mucus in the pancreas.

He argues that diseases cannot exist in an alkaline environment and when your body becomes too acidic.

By strictly following your diet and using your expensive supplements, it promises to restore your body's natural alkaline state and detoxify your sick body.

Originally, Dr. Sebi claimed it could cure diseases like AIDS, sickle cell anemia, leukemia, and lupus. However, after a 1993 lawsuit, he was ordered to cease making such claims.

The diet is a specific list of approved vegetables, fruits, grains, nuts, seeds, oils, and herbs. As animal products are not allowed, Dr. Sebi's diet is considered a vegan diet.

Sebi claimed you must be consistently on the diet for the rest of your life to heal your body.

Though many people insist that the program cure them, no scientific study supports these claims.

Dr. Sebi's diet emphasizes foods and supplements that are believed to decrease disease-causing mucus by reaching an alkaline state in your body.

8 Important Rules to Perfectly Follow the Dr. Sebi Diet

The rules of Dr. Sebi's diet are very strict and described on his website.

According to Dr. Sebi's nutritional guide, you need to follow these key rules:

- Rule 1. You should only eat the foods listed in the nutritional guide.
- Rule 2. Drink 1 gallon (3.8 liters) of water per day.
- Rule 3. Take Dr Sebi's supplements one hour before the medication.
- Rule 4. No products of animal origin are permitted.
- Rule 5. Alcohol is not permitted.
- Rule 6. Avoid wheat products and eat only the "naturally growing grains" listed in the guide.
- Rule 7. Avoid using a microwave oven to avoid killing your food.
- Rule 8. Avoid canned or seedless fruit.

No specific nutrient guidelines exist. This diet, however, is low in protein, prohibiting beans, lentils, animal products, and soy. Protein is an important nutrient for strong muscle, skin, and joints.

It is recommended to buy the "all-inclusive" package, which contains 20 different products that are supposed to cleanse and restore your entire body at the fastest rate possible.

Additionally, no specific supplement recommendation is provided. Rather, you are expected to order any supplement that matches your health concerns.

For example, "Bio Ferro" capsules claim to treat liver problems, purify the blood, boost immunity, promote weight loss, help digestive problems, and increase general well-being.

Additionally, supplements do not contain a complete list of nutrients or their amounts, making it difficult to know if they meet your daily needs.

Dr. Sebi's diet has eight main rules to follow. They focus on avoiding animal products, ultra-processed foods, and taking their proprietary supplements.

The cons of the Dr. Sebi diet

Keep in mind that there are several downsides to this diet.

Very restrictive

One of the main drawbacks to Dr Sebi's diet is that it restricts large food groups, such as all animal products, wheat, beans, lentils, and many types of vegetables and fruits.

It is so strict that it only allows certain types of fruit. For example, you can eat cherry or plum tomatoes, but not other varieties like steak or roma tomatoes.

Additionally, following such a restrictive diet is unpleasant. It can lead to a negative relationship with food, especially since this diet denigrates foods not listed in the nutrition guide.

Finally, this diet encourages other negative behaviors, such as using supplements to complete. Since supplements are not a major calorie source, this claim further promotes unhealthy eating habits.

Lack of protein and other essential nutrients

A great source of nutrition may be the foods listed in Dr. Sebi's nutrition guide.

None of the foods permitted, however, are a good source of protein, a nutrient essential for the structure of the skin, muscle growth, and enzyme and hormone production.

Only nuts, Brazilian nuts, sesame seeds, and cannabis seeds, not great sources of protein, are allowed. For example, 1/4 of a cup of nuts (25 grams) and 3 tbsp. 4 grams and 9 grams of protein provide 1 tablespoon (30 grams) of hemp seeds, respectively. You should eat very large portions of these foods to meet your daily protein requirements.

Although the foods on this diet are high in certain nutrients, such as beta-carotene, potassium, and vitamins C and E, they are low in omega-3s, iron, calcium, and vitamins D and B12, which are nutrients of common interest to people following a strictly plant-based diet.

Dr. Sebi's website states that some ingredients in his supplements are proprietary and are not listed. This is worrying, because it's not clear what nutrients you are consuming and how much, making it difficult to know if you will meet your daily nutrient needs.

Not based on real science

A major concern with Dr. Sebi's diet approach is the lack of scientific evidence to support it.

He claims the dietary foods and supplements control your body's acid production. However, the human body strictly regulates the acid-base balance to maintain blood pH between 7.36 and 7.44, making your body slightly alkaline.

In rare cases like diabetes ketoacidosis, blood pH may exceed this range. It can be fatal without medical attention.

Finally, research has shown that your diet can change your urine pH slightly and temporarily, but not blood ph. Therefore, following Dr. Sebi's diet will not make your body more alkaline.

Dr. Sebi's diet may promote weight loss, but it is very restrictive and low in several essential nutrients such as protein, omega-3s, iron, calcium, and D and B12 vitamins. It also ignores your body's ability to regulate blood ph.

CHAPTER 2: DOCTOR SEBI'S PROCEDURE TO EFFECTIVELY LOSE WEIGHT

A healthy dietary regime, according to his approach, makes it difficult for any disease to survive in the body. Dr. Sebi's method focuses on eliminating body mucus, best achieved through alkaline foods and plant-based diets.

His diet is based on over 40 years of research. This long herbalist and naturalist practice enabled him to identify the best healthy alkaline foods.

The diet for Dr. Sebi is vegan, so it is built around products based on animals. It goes one step further, however, its objective is to find the most natural foods to promote health and eliminate levels of body acid.

A diet rich in alkaline foods prevents the body from building up mucus, which is the main cause of illness, according to Dr. Sebi.

In Honduras, Dr. Sebi founded the USHA Healing Village. He has developed numerous dietary guides to help cure some illnesses, targeting individuals with particular diseases such as cancer.

His general dietary plan, however, is good for anyone who wants to focus on healthier living.

Dr. Sebi died in 2016, but his diet plan continues. Since different followers have tried to adjust Dr. Sebi's method differently.

Therefore, several variations and updates on Dr. Sebi's method can be found. The core of all these dietary approaches, however, is the same, based on Dr. Sebi's approach to food and well-being.

Dr. Sebi's diet focuses on alkaline food. According to Dr. Sebi, these foods can improve your health and well-being by reducing body acid content.

Reducing acid content in your body's foods and mucus promotes strength and health, including Dr. Sebi Diet Plan's main goals. Dr. Sebi recommends a vegan diet approach, rich in natural, plant-based foods.

Dr. Sebi Diet's plan is more than a program. It promotes a new food approach and lifestyle. This is not a quick-results diet plan.

It offers long-term dietary changes and promotes overall well-being. However, as this dietary regime eliminates sugar and processed foods, it leads to weight loss for those who use it.

According to Dr. Sebi, acidic foods can damage the body and should be avoided. His dietary approach emphasizes alkaline foods, promoting health and eliminating organism toxins.

Your diet should consist mostly of live and raw foods to stay healthy.

These foods are alkaline and from the dead and acidic foods will help heal your body. Meat, seafood, alcohol, and sugar are the primary acidic foods.

Synthetic and processed items are also considered acidic, as are fried foods. Keep in mind that the Dr. Sebi Diet Plan restricts all human-made, genetically modified, and hybrid foods.

Seedless fruits, insect-resistant, and weather-resistant crops are other foods that need to be avoided under Dr. Sebi's diet plan.

These include maize, certain types of tomatoes, as well as foods containing added minerals and vitamins. Instead, leafy greens, ripe fruit, non-starchy vegetables, and nuts are encouraged by this diet plan.

You are also permitted to eat certain grains from your diet, such as rye, quinoa, and Kamut, but minimize or eliminate the other grains.

Such a dietary regime is specifically designed to remove the body from toxins, waste, and acidic elements. You will lose weight and embrace a completely new approach to food by switching to an alkaline, plant-based diet.

Dr. Sebi Food List

The Dr. Sebi Diet Plan is a strictly vegan diet system focused on the entire diet based on food plants. It emphasizes foods that have been listed as alkaline by Dr Sebi.

This means that all plant-based foods are not allowed to be eaten (see below). All the foods that you eat while following this diet plan must be on the list of approved foods.

Here is a food list for Dr. Sebi with what you can eat on the diet plan for Dr. Sebi:

Vegetables:
- Green amaranth - like Callaloo, a variety of spinach
- Lawyer
- Asperges
- Peppers
- Banana Butter
- Chayote (Mexico squash)
- Cucumber
- Dandelion leaves
- Chickpeas (chickpeas) - optional
- Izote - cactus flower/cactus leaf - grows naturally in California

- ✓ Jicama
- ✓ Cabbage
- ✓ Lettuce (all except Iceberg)
- ✓ Mushrooms (all except Shitake)
- ✓ Mustard leaves
- ✓ Nopales - Mexican Cactus
- ✓ Okra
- ✓ Olives (and olive oil)
- ✓ Onions
- ✓ Green salads
- ✓ Sea vegetables (wakame / dulse / arame / hijiki / nori)
- ✓ Squash
- ✓ Spinach (use sparingly)
- ✓ Beans
- ✓ Tomato - cherry and plum only
- ✓ Tomatillo
- ✓ Turnip leaves
- ✓ Zucchini

Fruits:

- ✓ Pommes
- ✓ Bananas - the smallest or medium / Butter (original banana)
- ✓ Berries - all varieties of elderberries - in any form - without cranberries
- ✓ Cantaloupe
- ✓ Cherries
- ✓ Currant
- ✓ At your place
- ✓ figs
- ✓ Grape-seeds
- ✓ Limes (favorite key files with seeds)
- ✓ Mango
- ✓ Melons-seeds
- ✓ Orange (Seville or favorite bitter, hard to find)
- ✓ Papaya
- ✓ Peaches
- ✓ Pears
- ✓ Plums

- ✓ Grape-seeds
- ✓ Sweet coconut jelly (and coconut oil)
- ✓ Carousels -Latin or West Indian markets)
- ✓ Sugary apples (from cherimoya)

Nuts and seeds:

- ✓ Prime almonds and almond butter
- ✓ Raw sesame seeds
- ✓ "Tahini" with raw sesame butter
- ✓ Nuts / hazelnuts

Spices – seasonings:

- ✓ Achiote
- ✓ Basil
- ✓ Bay leaf
- ✓ Cayenne
- ✓ Coriander
- ✓ Coriander
- ✓ Cumin
- ✓ Dill
- ✓ Marjoram
- ✓ Onion powder
- ✓ Origin
- ✓ Granulated seaweed powder (seaweed / Dulce / Nori - tastes like the sea ")
- ✓ Pure sea salt
- ✓ Sage
- ✓ Sweet basil
- ✓ Tarragon
- ✓ Thyme

Sugars:

- ✓ 100% pure agave syrup - (from cactus)
- ✓ Date "sugar" (from dry dates)
- ✓ 100% Pure Maple Syrup - Grade B recommended
- ✓ Maple "Sugar" (from dried maple syrup)
- ✓ Nutritional Guide | Alkaline grains
- ✓ Amar ante

- ✓ Black rice
- ✓ Kamut
- ✓ Quinoa
- ✓ Rye
- ✓ Spelled
- ✓ Tef
- ✓ Wild rice

All-natural herbal teas:

- ✓ Albahaca
- ✓ Anise
- ✓ Chamomile
- ✓ Clove
- ✓ Fennel
- ✓ Ginger
- ✓ Lemongrass
- ✓ Raspberry red
- ✓ Sea moss tea
- ✓ Alkaline Diet - Herbs to cleanse and revitalize my organs
- ✓ Burdock root - cleanser for blood and liver, diuretic,
- ✓ Bladderwrack (seaweed) - vitamins and mineral supplements
- ✓ The black walnut is killing pests
- ✓ Bromelain and papain: dissolves proteins in the small intestine
- ✓ Chlorella (algae) - protein, vitamins, and mineral supplements, detoxifying
- ✓ Curcumin - antioxidant, supports brain, cardiovascular and joint health
- ✓ Dandelion - blood and liver cleanser
- ✓ Elderberry (Sambucus nigra) - strengthens the body against colds
- ✓ Flaxseed - fights heart disease, cancer, diabetes, high essential fatty acids
- ✓ Irish Moss (seaweed) - vitamins and mineral supplements
- ✓ Kelp (seaweed) - vitamins and mineral supplements
- ✓ Mullein - removes mucus from the small intestine
- ✓ Oregano oil - antiviral
- ✓ Sarsaparilla - blood purifier, diuretic, antibacterial, anti-inflammatory
- ✓ Wormwood Leaf - kills parasites

Oils:

- ✓ Olive oil (do not cook)

- ✓ Coconut oil (do not cook)
- ✓ Grapeseed oil (added)
- ✓ Sesame oil (added)
- ✓ Hemp oil (added)
- ✓ Avocado oil (added)

Foods to Avoid

All foods that are not included in the Dr. Sebi nutritional guide are not permitted, such as:

- ✗ Canned fruits or vegetables
- ✗ Seedless fruit
- ✗ Ova
- ✗ Dairy
- ✗ Fish
- ✗ Red meat
- ✗ Poultry
- ✗ Soy products
- ✗ Processed foods, including take out or restaurant foods
- ✗ Fortified foods
- ✗ Wheat
- ✗ Sugar (apart from date sugar and agave syrup)
- ✗ Alcohol
- ✗ Yeast or foods leavened with yeast
- ✗ Foods made with baking powder

Besides, many vegetables, fruits, grains, nuts, and seeds are prohibited in the diet. Only the foods listed in the guide can be eaten.

CHAPTER 3: DOCTOR SEBI DIET'S BENEFITS

One advantage of Dr the Sebi Diet is a heavy emphasis on plant foods.

The diet encourages the consumption of large numbers of vegetables and fruits rich in fiber, vitamins, minerals, and phytochemicals.

Diets high in vegetables and fruits have been linked to reducing inflammation and oxidative stress and protecting against many diseases.

In a study of 65,226 people, those who ate 7 or more servings of vegetables and fruits per day had a 25% and 31% lower incidence of cancer and heart disease, respectively.

Moreover, most people do not eat enough. In a 2017 report, 9.3% and 12.2% respectively met recommendations for vegetables and fruits.

Besides, the Dr Sebi diet includes high-fiber whole grain products and healthy fats such as nuts, seeds, and vegetable oils. These foods were linked to lower heart disease risk.

Finally, diets that limit ultra-processed foods are linked to better overall diet quality.

Summary the Dr. Sebi Diet focuses on eating nutrient-dense vegetables, fruits, whole grains, and healthy fats, which can reduce the risk of heart disease, cancer, and inflammation.

Dr. Sebi Diet's 7-Day Meal Plan (Alkaline Diet Plan)

SAMPLE MENU

Here's a sample three-day menu on the Dr. Sebi diet.

Day 1

- **Breakfast:** 2 pancakes with banana spelled and agave syrup.
- **Snack I:** 1 cup (240 ml) green juice smoothie made from cucumber, kale, apples, and ginger.
- **Lunch:** kale salad with tomatoes, onions, avocado, dandelions, and chickpeas with olive oil and basil dressing.
- **Snack II:** herbal tea with fruits.
- **Dinner:** stir-fry vegetables and wild rice.

Day 2

- **Breakfast:** shake with water, hemp seeds, bananas, and strawberries.
- **Snack I:** blueberry muffins made from blueberries, pure coconut milk, agave syrup, sea salt, oil as well as teff and spelled flour.
- **Lunch:** homemade pizza with a spelled crust, Brazil nut cheese, and vegetables of your choice.

- **Snack II:** tahini butter on rye bread with sliced red peppers on the side.
- **Dinner:** chickpea burger with tomatoes, onions, and kale on spelled flour flatbread.

Day 3

- **Breakfast:** cooked quinoa with agave syrup, peaches, and pure coconut milk.
- **Snack I:** chamomile tea, grape seeds, and sesame seeds.
- **Lunch:** spelled pasta salad with chopped vegetables and olive oil and lime dressing.
- **Snack II:** a smoothie made from mango, banana, and pure coconut milk.
- **Dinner:** hearty vegetable soup with mushrooms, peppers, zucchini, onions, kale, spices, water, and seaweed powder.

Day 4

- **Breakfast:** cooked quinoa with agave syrup, peaches, and pure coconut milk.
- **Snack I:** chamomile tea, grape seeds, and sesame seeds.
- **Lunch:** spelled pasta salad with chopped vegetables and olive oil and lime dressing.
- **Snack II:** a smoothie made from mango, banana, and pure coconut milk.
- **Dinner:** hearty vegetable soup with mushrooms, peppers, zucchini, onions, kale, spices, water, and seaweed powder.

Day 5

- **Breakfast:** shake with water, hemp seeds, bananas, and strawberries.
- **Snack I:** blueberry muffins made from blueberries, pure coconut milk, agave syrup, sea salt, oil as well as teff and spelled flour.
- **Lunch:** homemade pizza with a spelled crust, Brazil nut cheese, and vegetables of your choice.
- **Snack II:** tahini butter on rye bread with sliced red peppers on the side.
- **Dinner:** chickpea burger with tomatoes, onions, and kale on spelled flour flatbread.

Day 6

- **Breakfast:** 1 glass of chlorophyll juice. Preparation: In a blender, mix 2 cabbage leaves, 1 cup (tea) of watercress leaves, 1 lettuce or fennel leaf, 1 glass of pure orange juice, 1/2 grated carrot, a handful of mint, or 1 tablespoon watercress. Minced ginger. Sweetener and ice to taste.
- **Lunch:** 1 plate with green salad: lettuce, chard, raw cabbage, onion, spring onion, celery and mushroom, 4 col. (Chickpea soup, 2 col. Shredded chicken (soup).
- **Snack:** 2 handfuls of toasted sunflower or pumpkin seeds, 1 Chickpea paste grain soup celery + + + yellow pepper tomatoes, 1 tangerine.

- **Dinner:** 2 plates of vegetable soup with kombu seaweed and 2 cabbage. (Soup) of wild or whole rice or 2 plates of pumpkin soup with kombu seaweed (alkaline and rich in minerals).

Day 7

- **Breakfast:** 2 pancakes with banana spelled and agave syrup.
- **Snack I:** 1 cup (240 ml) green juice smoothie made from cucumber, kale, apples, and ginger.
- **Lunch:** kale salad with tomatoes, onions, avocado, dandelions, and chickpeas with olive oil and basil dressing.
- **Snack II:** herbal tea with fruits.
- **Dinner:** stir-fry vegetables and wild rice.

This sample meal plan emphasizes the approved ingredients included in the Food Nutrition Guide. The meals in this plan emphasize vegetables and fruits with small amounts from the other food groups.

The Dr. Sebi diet promotes the consumption of whole, unprocessed, plant-based foods.

It can help with weight loss if you don't eat normally that way.

It depends heavily, however, on taking costly designer supplements, is very restrictive, lacks certain nutrients, and promises inaccurately to change your body to an alkaline state.

A lot of healthy diets are more flexible and sustainable if you are looking to adopt a more plant-based diet.

Frequently Asked Questions

- ➢ **Can anyone start a Dr Sebi alkaline diet?**
- For the most part, yes. The diet is suitable for any adult who wants to detoxify their body or prevent problems. Those suffering from chronic digestive disorders, skin problems, allergies, migraines or rheumatism can benefit from an alkaline diet.

- ➢ **Is the Dr Sebi alkaline diet suitable for vegans?**
- There is absolutely yes! For a healthier lifestyle, more and more individuals opt for plant-based diets, and the diet is no exception. Do not forget to mention that when you book your hotel, you are vegan to inform the hotel before your arrival.

- ➢ **What foods can I eat on Dr Sebi alkaline diet?**
- In addition to the abundance of water and herbal teas, all foods with an alkalizing effect are eaten. In other words:
- Almost all types of vegetables (including potatoes), herbs, and salads
- All types of fruit (including dried fruit)
- Walnuts and hazelnuts

- Cold-pressed oils (belong to neutral foods)
- Besides, about four hours should elapse between meals to allow the digestive system to recover.

> **How long should I be on a Dr Sebi alkaline diet?**
- Alkaline fasting should be done for about a week or two. An alkaline surplus is recommended but not a purely alkaline diet, as there are also "good" acidifying foods that contribute to a healthy and lasting balance.

> **Which foods are "good" acidifiers?**
- Whole grains, brown rice, whole wheat bread, legumes are the "good" acidifiers. They generally contribute to a healthy body balance of alkalis and acids, though they should be avoided during an alkaline diet. They should be replenished after detoxification.

> **What are the benefits of a Dr Sebi alkaline diet?**
- The greatest advantage is probably that you can eat your fill. This makes the diet easy to follow and, without feeling sluggish, you can explore the most beautiful resorts. Your mood will also thank you. Another benefit is that, during this kind of fast, you provide your body with all the important nutrients. Cells and blood vessels are held in shape by vitamins, minerals, enzymes, and bioactive substances. Integrate what you have learned into your daily life once you return home and help prevent the allergies and illnesses of modern civilization. Dr Sebi diet also provides the basis for well-being and overall better health.

> **What are the possible side effects of a Dr Sebi alkaline diet?**
- Headache, dizziness, weakness, tiredness, sleeplessness, unpleasant body odor, problems with the skin. These are typical fasting side effects, which you fortunately do not have to worry about on an alkaline diet, because from now on you do not have to give up food completely! Heavy coffee drinkers may experience headaches initially, but after a day or two and no later than after a walk in the fresh air (in nature or along the seafront) they should disappear very quickly.

> **Can Dr Sebi alkaline diet help me lose weight?**
- Weight loss is not the goal of a Dr Sebi alkaline diet, but it can be a natural side effect. With an alkaline diet, you provide fewer calories than your body needs, and you avoid products like ready-to-use foods and simple sugars.

CHAPTER 4: BREAKFAST RECIPES

1. Spelled bread without yeast

Ingredients For 1 portion:

- 500 g spelled flour, type 630
- ½ TL salt
- ½ liter water, lukewarm
- 1 teaspoon bread spice mix
- 1 pck. cream of tartar
- 100 g linseed
- 100 g pumpkin seeds
- Olive oil for the baking dish

Preparation:

Working time approx. 10 minutes

Cooking/baking time approx. 1 hour

Total time approx. 1 hour 10 minutes

1. Mix the flour with the tartar powder. Then mix in salt, bread spice, flax seeds, and pumpkin seeds. Finally, add the lukewarm water and knead by hand.
2. Grease a box mold with a little olive oil and fill in the dough. Brushing the surface of the dough with a little water will make it nice and crispy.
3. Place in the cold oven and bake at 200 ° C top/bottom heat for 60 minutes.
4. The same dough can also be used for delicious spelled rolls eg with sunflower seeds.

2. Puff pastry - quiche with broccoli and camembert

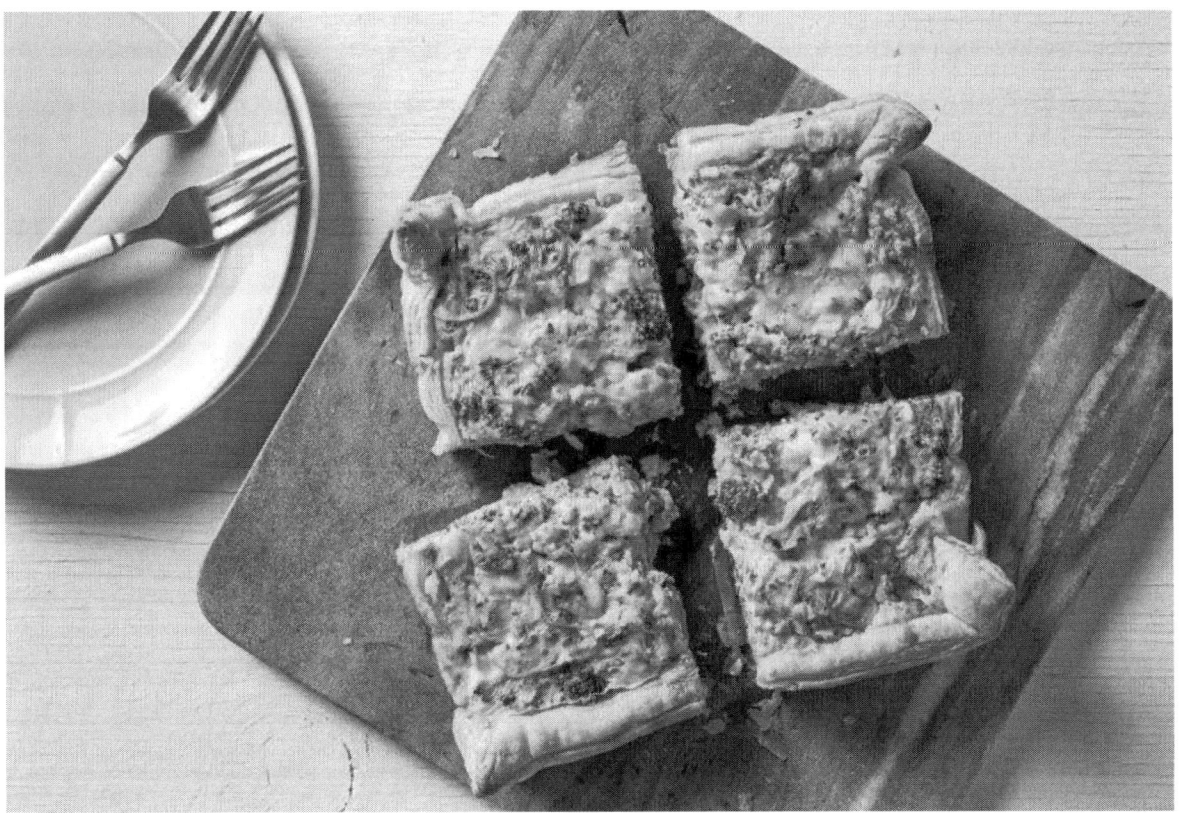

Ingredients For 6 portions:

- 1 pck. puff pastry from the refrigerated shelf
- 600g   broccoli or cauliflower, chard or spinach
- 200g   camembert
- 200ml cream
- 1 pinch nutmeg
- 2 egg
- Salt and pepper

Preparation:

Working time approx. 1 hour

Total time approx. 1 hour

1. Lay out the puff pastry in a springform pan. Preheat the oven to 180 ° C convection. Wash the broccoli and cut into small florets.
2. Put some water in a saucepan, add the broccoli and cook for about 5 minutes over medium heat. Drain in a sieve, drain and distribute on the dough. Cut the cheese into thin slices and decoratively lay on the broccoli.

3. Whisk the cream with eggs and spices and pour over the broccoli and cheese. Then bake on the middle rail for about 40 - 45 minutes golden yellow.
4. If you like, you can replace the broccoli with other vegetables (eg fresh leaf spinach - but then 1 kg, chard, or cauliflower). If you do not like camembert, you can also take feta cheese, then the quiche gets a very different note and the dish is nevertheless very basic. This fits a basic salad with lemon dressing.

3. Muesli basic mix

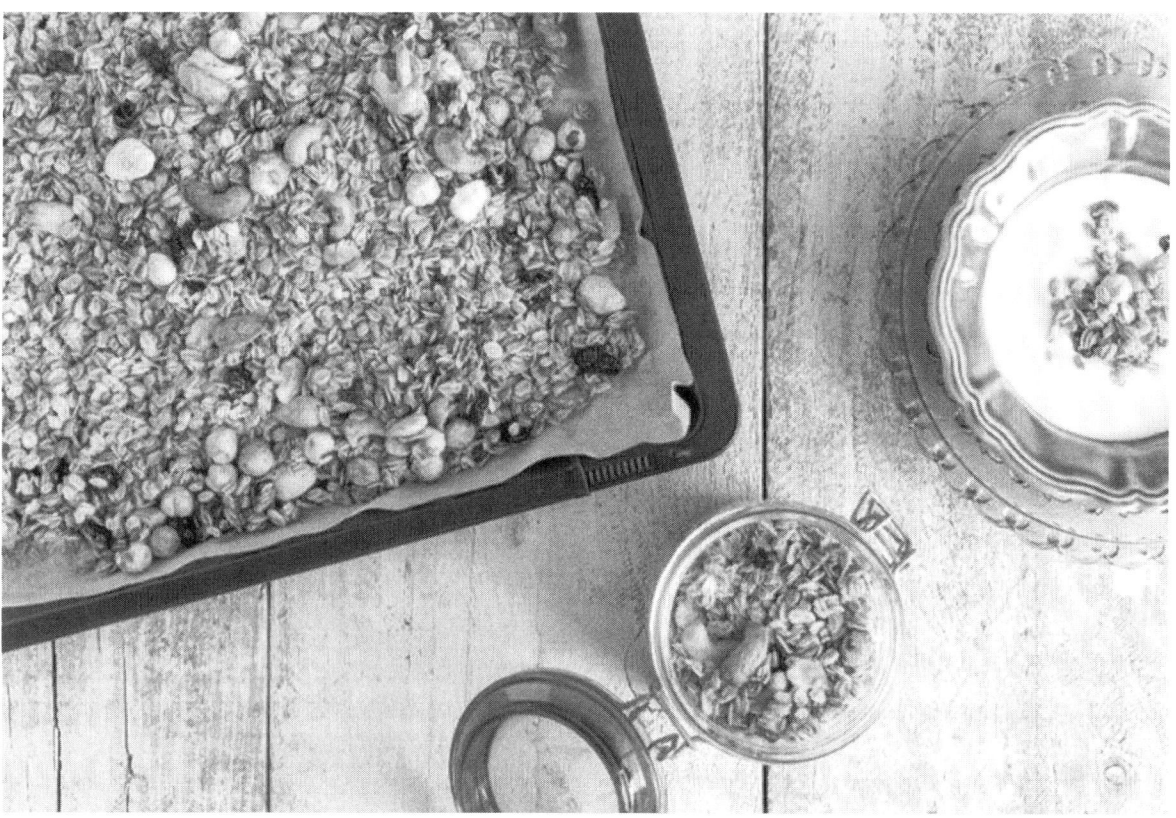

Ingredients For 1 portion:

- 20 g sugar, brown
- 70 g honey
- 2 teaspoons sesame oil
- ½ vanilla pod
- 1 teaspoon ground cinnamon
- 250 g oatmeal
- 20 g sesame
- 50 g almond (s), chopped
- 50 g almond (s), planed
- 50 g sunflower seeds

Preparation:

Working time approx. 20 minutes

Cooking/baking time approx. 15 minutes

Total time approx. 35 minutes

1. Scrape out the vanilla pod. In a large saucepan, heat sugar, honey, sesame oil, cinnamon, and the pith of the vanilla pod together with the vanilla pod at low temperature until the sugar has melted. Remove the vanilla pod. Evenly submerge the oatmeal, sesame seeds, and sunflower seeds. This may take a little longer, but stir, again and again, toss the sugar from the wooden spoon and fold again until everything is well mixed. Spread the mixture on a baking sheet lined with baking paper, place in the oven, and bake at 175 ° C for approx. 7 minutes, depending on the type of stovetop. Sprinkle the chopped and sliced almonds over and bake for about 7 minutes until the mass becomes slightly brownish and smells pleasant.
2. Allow to cool on the tin and place it in a tin.
3. If necessary, mix with yogurt and dried or fresh fruit.

4. Spelled bread with sunflower seeds

Ingredients For 1 portion:

- 500 g spelled flour, type 1050
- 250 g spelled flour, type 630
- ½ tbsp. salt
- ¾ liter water, lukewarm
- 250 g sunflower seeds, or others
- 1 teaspoon bread spice mix
- 2 pck. cream of tartar
- Oil (coconut), or other oil, for the mold

Preparation:

Working time approx. 10 minutes

Cooking/baking time approx. 45 minutes

Total time approx. 55 minutes

1. First mix all dry ingredients and then pour in the lukewarm water, knead well with dough hook.
2. Please do not be surprised, the dough is looser (tough-tearing) than usual.
3. Grease a box mold. Pour in dough, dab the dough surface with a little water to make the crust nice and crispy.

4. Bake in the preheated oven at 200 degrees for 30 minutes. During the first 30 min. slide on the middle rail and for the last 15 min. on the lowest, so that the bread is not too dark.
5. Since I have a small baking dish, I fill the remaining dough in Muffinförmchen and have it in 25 min. super delicious, freshly baked small rolls.

5. Fruit buckwheat porridge with pomegranate seeds

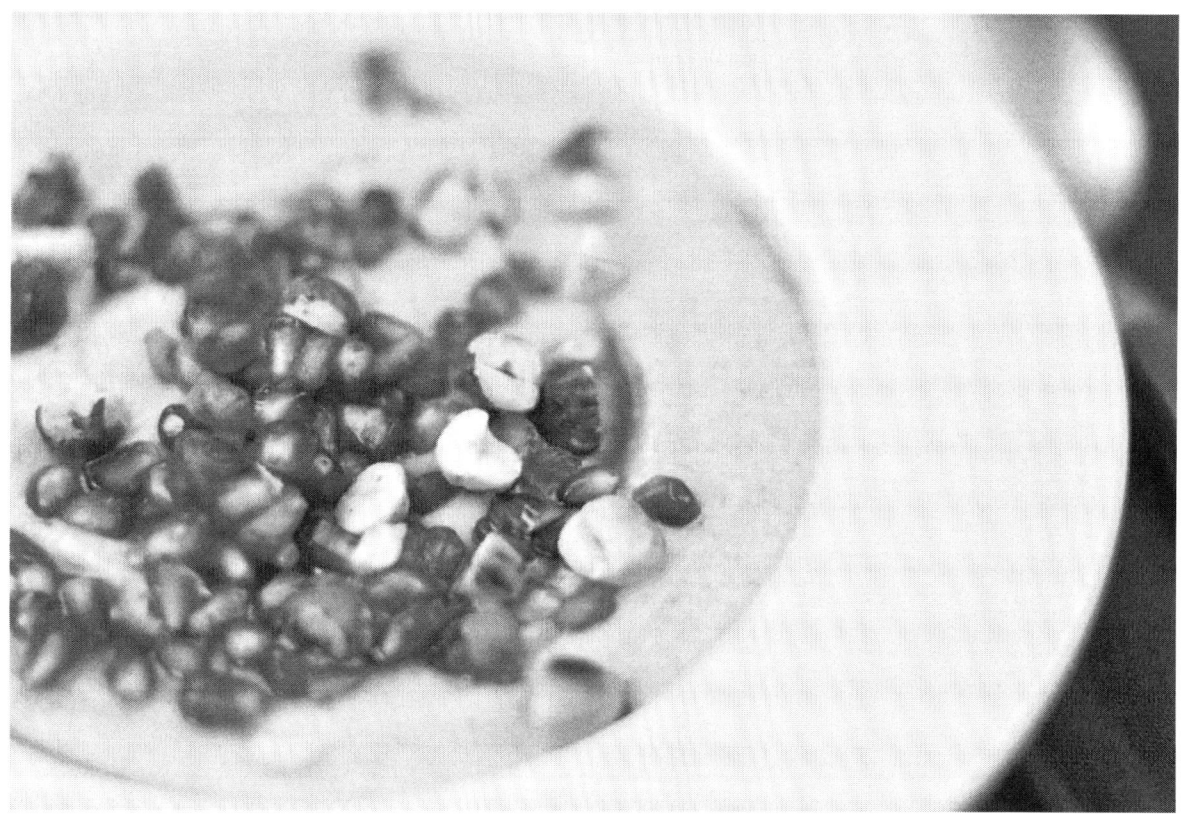

Ingredients For 2 portions:

- 100 g buckwheat
- 2 bulbs
- Banana
- Apple
- 1 handful raisins
- 2 teaspoons sweet lupine flour, optional
- 2 teaspoons almond butter
- 2 teaspoons lemon juice
- 100 ml almond milk (almond drink)
- Pomegranate

Preparation:

Working time approx. 20 minutes

Resting time approx. 2 days

Cooking/baking time approx. 4 hours

Total time approx. 2 days 4 hours 20 minutes

1. Soak the buckwheat in water for 1 hr, pour into a colander, rinse off and allow to stand in the colander over a bowl to germinate, rinsing under running water in the morning and evening. Buckwheat germinates after 1 - 2 days (it is then alkaline, has more nutrients, and is more compatible) and can be further processed.
2. Distribute 3 - 4 tablespoons of germinated buckwheat on a baking sheet and let it circulate in the oven at approx. 50 ° C circulating air for approx. 3 - 4 hours. If you have a dehydrator, of course, you better take this.
3. Add the remaining buckwheat to the blender with raisins, sweet lupine flour, almond paste, lemon juice, and almond milk. Core the pears and apple. Peel the banana. Add the fruit as well. Everything about 90 sec. Mix well. If the porridge is too firm, add some almond milk, but not too much, it should not be liquid.
4. Distribute the fruit pulp into two cereal bowls.
5. Remove the pomegranates from the pomegranate and add to the ingredients. Allow the dried buckwheat grains to cool slightly and then distribute them on top.

6. Buckwheat semolina

Ingredients For 2 portions:

- 400 ml coconut milk
- 200 ml almond milk (almond drink), unsweetened
- 100 g semolina (buckwheat semolina)
- 1 handful fruit of choice, fresh

Preparation:

Working time approx. 15 minutes

Total time approx. 15 minutes

1. Boil the coconut and almond milk in a saucepan. Remove the pot from the heat and stir in the buckwheat semolina.
2. Fill the semolina pudding into dessert bowls, allow to cool slightly, and enjoy with fresh fruit.

7. Maroni coconut cream "Symphony of the trees"

Ingredients For 1 portion:

- 2 tbsp chestnut flour or chestnut raw food powder
- 100 ml coconut milk, up to 200 ml
- 1 shot water
- 1 pinch salt
- 1 tbsp almond butter
- 1 handful fruit, cut small, depending on the season
- 1 teaspoon cinnamon

Preparation:

Working time approx. 15 minutes

Total time approx. 15 minutes

1. Strain the chestnut raw food powder/flour with a dash of water and salt. If you prefer the ayurvedic variant, this can still heat up.
2. Put this porridge on a deep plate, add warm coconut milk (about 100 - 200 ml), and cut fruit. On top of that, almond paste and cinnamon.

8. Dark chocolate cream with figs

Ingredients For 1 portion:

- 50 g fig (s), dried
- 25 ml water
- ground cinnamon
- 5 g cocoa powder, slightly de-oiled
- 10 g cream

Preparation:

Working time approx. 5 minutes

Rest time approx. 1 hour

Total time approx. 1 hour 5 minutes

1. Chop the figs very small and add half as much water, in this case, 25 ml. Stir well and leave to soak for an hour.
2. Now add the cocoa powder, the cinnamon at will, and the cream and stir well.
3. I like to eat this cream on bread or in pancakes.

4   This recipe can also be varied in many ways. Instead of figs, take dried dates, vanilla pods, or ground nuts.

9. Apple and coconut cream

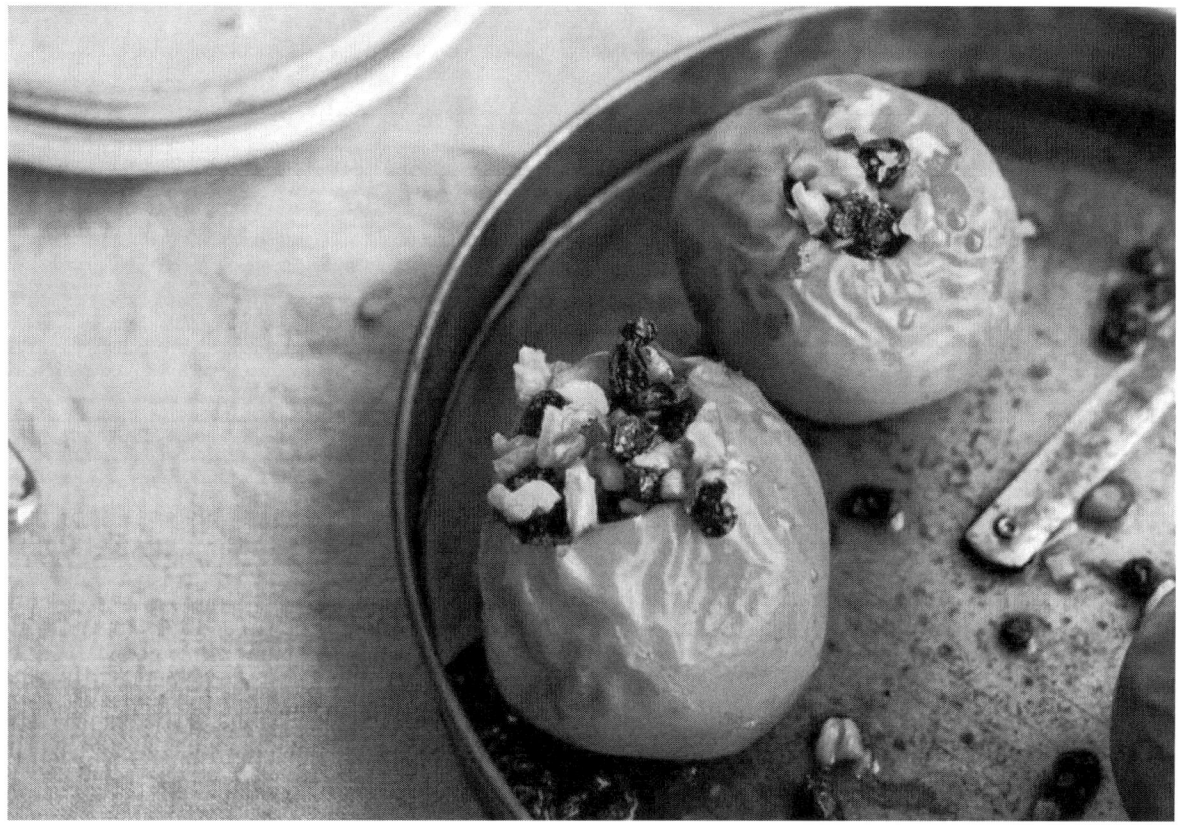

Ingredients For 2 portions:

- 360 g apple pulp
- 4 TL, heaped brown millet, ground
- 2 tablespoons, heaped gingernut flakes
- 1 teaspoon cinnamon
- 1 tbsp lemon juice
- 250 g yogurt (coconut milk yogurt), vegan, gluten-free

Preparation:

Working time approx. 5 minutes

Total time approx. 5 minutes

- Put all ingredients in a bowl and stir.

10. Apple and almond muesli mandarins

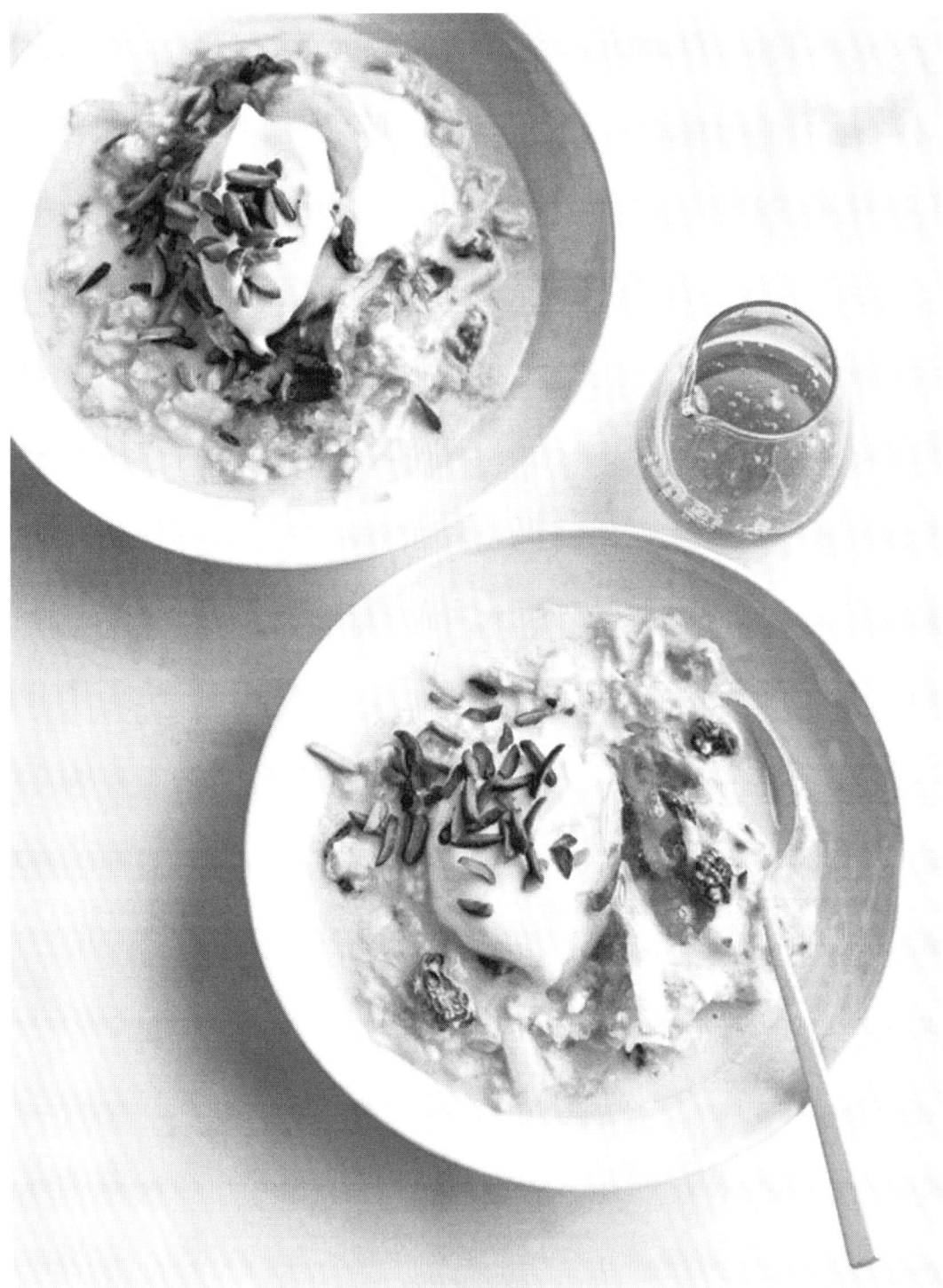

Ingredients For 2 portions:

- Apples
- 2 tbsp almond, planed
- 3 tbsp walnuts, chopped

- 2 tbsp tigernut (tigernut chufas nüssli)
- 2 tbsp cranberries
- Mandarine

Preparation:

Working time approx. 10 minutes

Total time approx. 10 minutes

- Squeeze out the tangerines and put the juice in a bowl. Peel, quarter, core and grate the apples, add to the juice, and stir. Add almonds, walnuts, Chufas-Nüssli, and cranberries.

11. Danny's morning hour - basic breakfast buffet

Ingredients For 2 Portions:

- 1 tbsp millet, or double the amount already popped or ground, see instructions
- 1 tbsp buckwheat, or twice the amount already popped or ground, see instructions
- 250 ml almond milk (almond drink) or oat milk (oat drink)
- 1 tbsp amaranth, puffed or half puffed and then puffed yourself, see instructions
- 1 tbsp sunflower seeds
- 1 tbsp pumpkin seeds
- 1 tbsp almond (s), whole
- 1 apple
- 2 tbsp pineapple pieces, frozen

Preparation:

Working time approx. 10 minutes

Cooking/baking time approx. 3 minutes

Total time approx. 13 minutes

1. Put 2 tablespoons of millet and buckwheat into a flaker or a flour mill and flake or grind. I always use the Flocker. Those who do not have both should buy flakes in the organic market. It then takes about twice the amount as flakes.
2. Put in a saucepan 250 ml of almond milk or similar liquid that you like. In the cold liquid stir the flakes. Bring the almond milk to a boil while stirring and stir until the porridge has the desired consistency. This usually takes only 1 - 2 minutes. Remove the pot from the heat and add the tablespoon of popped Amaranth. A good blender (for smoothies) puree the chopped apple, the frozen pineapple pieces, the sunflower and pumpkin seeds, and almonds with a dash of water. Stir the mixture into the porridge.

12. Basic breakfast buffet with buckwheat

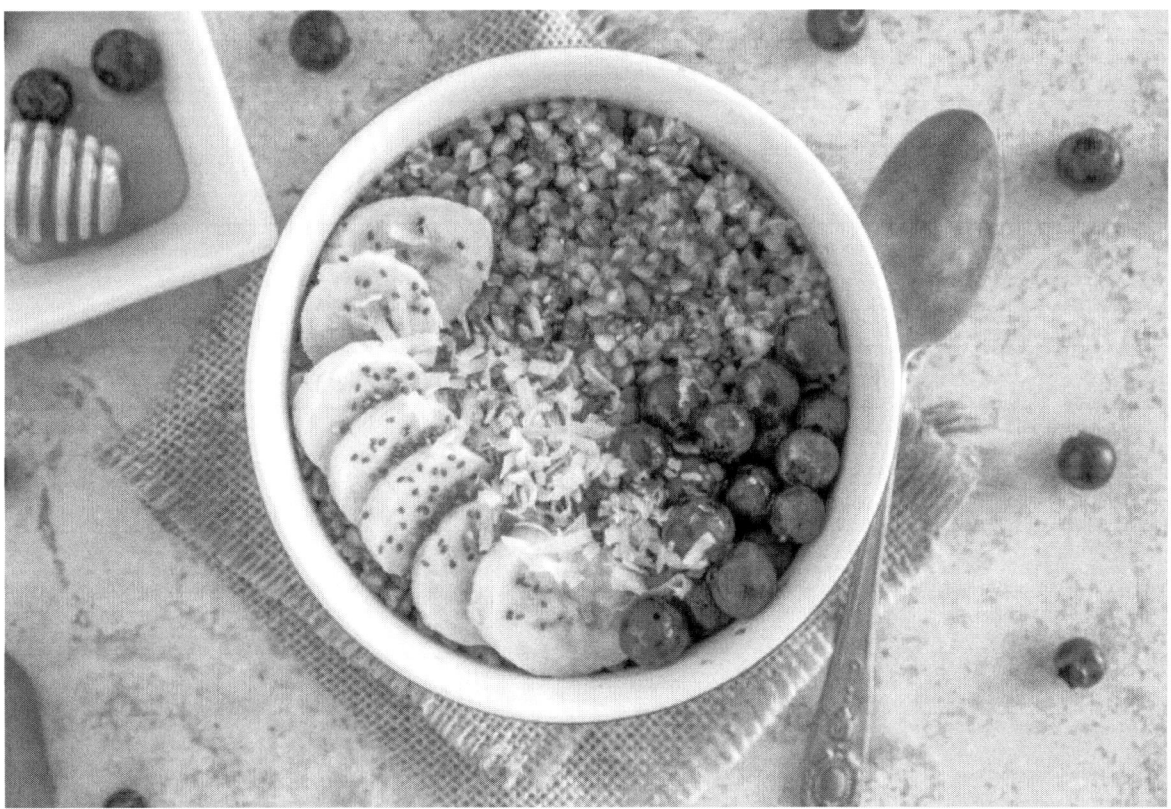

Ingredients For 2 people:

- Organic apple 2 pieces / 200g
- Carrots 2 pieces / 120g
- Banana / n 1 piece / 110g
- Buckwheat flour 50 grams
- Water 400 grams
- Rapeseed oil (native) 1 tablespoon / 12g
- Walnuts 3 tablespoons / 30g
- Salt 1 pinch / n / 1g

Preparation:

1. Bring water to a boil with a pinch of salt. Wash buckwheat semolina with hot running water in a strainer. Remove the pot from the heat, add the buckwheat semolina and simmer over low heat while stirring for about 5 minutes.
2. In the meantime, wash the carrots and apple, peel and finely grate. Crush banana. Anyone who wants to can puree everything together with the oil.

3. Stir fruit-carrot mixture and the oil in the still warm breakfast porridge. Fill the basic breakfast porridge with buckwheat semolina into two small bowls and serve. Bon Appetit!

13. Basic cereal

Ingredients For 2 people:

- Millet grains 20 grams
- Buckwheat 50 grams
- Pumpkin seeds 30 grams
- Sunflower seeds 30 grams
- Hazelnuts 30 grams
- Date 3 pieces / 15g
- Organic apple 1 piece / 120g
- Cinnamon something / 1g
- Water 400 grams

Preparation:

1. Crush buckwheat, millet, seeds, and nuts with a suitable kitchen appliance, eg a powerful smoothie maker.
2. Cut the dates and the fig into the smallest possible pieces.
3. Bring all shredded basic foods to a boil with approx. 400 ml of water and turn the temperature down for 3 minutes.
4. In the meantime, peel an apple or another basic fruit (eg banana) and peel it into bite-sized pieces.
5. Remove the basic muesli from the heat, cool slightly, stir in apple and cinnamon and serve. Bon Appetit!

Note: The basic muesli can also be prepared in advance for simply preparing larger quantities without fresh fruit and keeping them airtight. The basic muesli mixture lasts for several weeks.

Nutritional information:

	per 100g	per serving
Kilojoules (calories)	1808 (432)	520 (124)
Protein	15.45 g	4.44 g
Carbohydrates	44.43 g	12.77 g

Fat	21.27 g	6.11 g
Fructose	11.10 g	3.19 g
Sorbitol	0.25 g	0.07 g
Glucose	8.43 g	2.42 g
Lactose content	0.00 g	0.00 g

14. Fruit salad with strawberries and tigernuts

Ingredients For 4 people:

- Apples 2 pieces / 220g
- Strawberries 250 grams
- Blueberries 80 grams
- Kiwi /s 2 pieces / 160g
- Orange juice 150 milliliters
- Orange / 1 piece / 150g
- Gingernuts flakes 200 grams

Preparation:

1. Peel the apples and prepare on a grater in small pieces or Mus. Chop the remaining fruit and put everything in a bowl.
2. Mix the orange juice with the Chufas Nüssli (strawberry flakes) and let it swell briefly. Then combine everything.
3. A purely basic breakfast!

15. Oatmeal Seasoned with Vegetables

What you will need:

- 4 cups of water
- 2 cups of "cut" oatmeal (quick-cooking steel-cut oats)
- 1 teaspoon Italian spices
- ½ teaspoon Herbamare or sea salt
- 1 teaspoon garlic powder
- 1 teaspoon onion powder

- ½ cup nutritional yeast
- ¼ teaspoon turmeric powder
- 1½ cup kale or tender spinach
- ½ cup sliced mushrooms
- ¼ cup grated carrots
- ½ cup small chopped peppers

Process:

1. Boil the water in a saucepan.
2. Add the oatmeal and spices and lower the temperature.
3. Cook over low heat without lid for 5 to 7 minutes.
4. Add the vegetables.
5. Cover and set aside for 2 minutes.
6. Serve immediately.

16. Blackberry and lemon muffins for tea

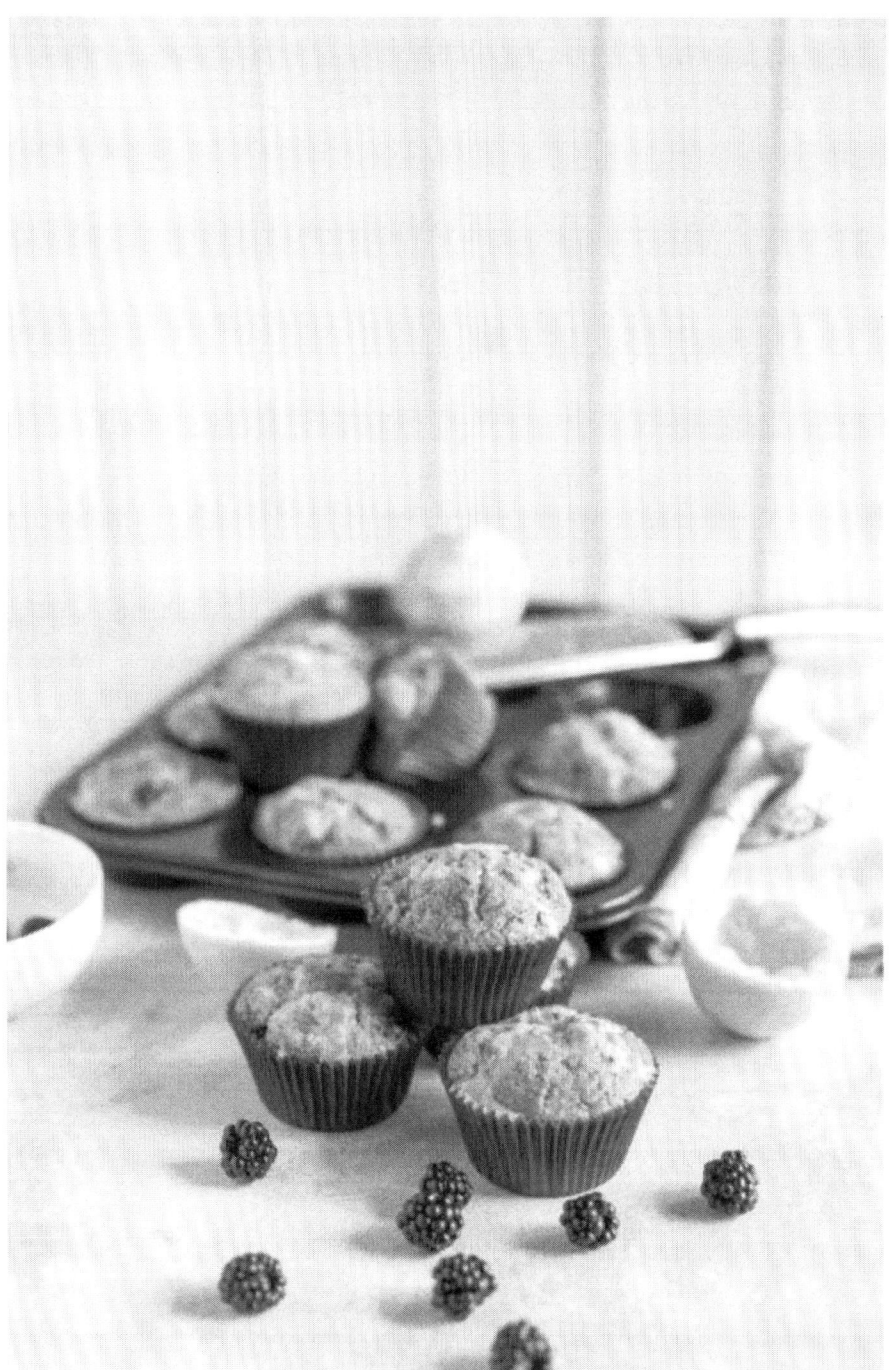

What you will need:

- 2 cups whole grain wheat flour for baking
- ½ cup of Sucanat (refined cane sugar)
- 1½ teaspoon baking powder
- 1 teaspoon grated lemon peel
- ½ cup natural soy yogurt

- 1 cup non-dairy milk
- 1 tablespoon lemon juice
- 2 egg substitutes (2 tablespoons ground flaxseed with 6 tablespoons water)
- 1 cup blackberries
- 2 tablespoons coconut with reduced-fat and sugar-free content (optional)

Process:

1. Preheat to 350 ° F (177 ° C) in the oven.
2. Fill a paper-coated mold for 12 muffins (or use a non-stick skillet).
3. In a medium bowl, mix flour, sucanat sweetener, baking powder, and rubbed lemon peel.
4. In a separate bowl, mix soy yogurt, milk, lemon juice, and egg substitutes.
5. Pour into the dry mixture the wet mixture and stir until it is hot.
6. Carefully add blackberries.
7. In the prepared muffin pan, distribute the mixture evenly.
8. Sprinkle the coconut (optional) on top of the muffins.
9. Bake them for 45 minutes in the preheated oven or until one of them has a toothpick inserted in the middle. Until serving, let them cool slightly.

17. Cherry and poppy seed muffins

What you will need:

DRY

- 1 cup (120 g) raw buckwheat flour
- 1 ¼ cup oatmeal (155 g) oatmeal
- 2 tablespoons poppy seeds
- 2 teaspoons cinnamon
- ½ teaspoon cardamom
- 2 teaspoons baking powder

WET

- 10 chopped figs
- A little more than 1 cup (260 ml) of vegetable milk, without sugar
- 2 ripe bananas
- 2 heaped tablespoons unsweetened applesauce
- 2 tablespoons peanut butter
- 1 pinch of sea salt (optional)
- ½ cup (50 g) dark chocolate (at least 70% cocoa), chopped

- 24 fresh or frozen cherries

Process:

1. Preheat the oven to 180 ° C (355 ° F).
2. Cut the figs and soak them in vegetable milk for at least 30 minutes. If you want to dip it further, put it in the refrigerator.
3. While the figs are soaked, chop the chocolate and place it aside. Put all other dry ingredients in a bowl. Put the figs and milk into the mixer. Add all remaining wet ingredients and mix until smooth.
4. Pour the wet mixture over the dry ingredients and mix well. Make sure there are no lumps. Add chopped chocolate.
5. The mold is filled with 12 muffins (molded using silicon) with a lump and finally hits two cherries in each muffin.
6. Bake for 25-30 minutes. Allow it to cool a little before trying to remove it from the mold.

18. Cocoa, banana, and whole-grain spelled flour muffins

What you will need:

- 2 large bananas (I use frozen bananas and then defrost them)
- 2 cups whole grain spelled flour
- 1 cup walnuts, chopped into large pieces
- ½ cup raw cocoa powder
- ¼ cup applesauce
- 1 cup almond milk
- ¼ cup maple syrup, 100% pure
- ½ teaspoon baking powder

Process:

1. Preheat the oven to 300-350 ° F (177 ° C).
2. Line the muffin pan with baking paper.
3. Crush the bananas in a large bowl.
4. Add the almond milk, maple syrup, applesauce, and mix them.
5. Add whole-grain spelled flour, baking powder, and cocoa powder and mix them.
6. Add the chopped walnuts.
7. Pour the mixture into muffin pans.
8. Cook the muffins for about 25 minutes or until when a skewer is inserted, it is clean.

CHAPTER 5: SNACK RECIPES

19. Homemade granola

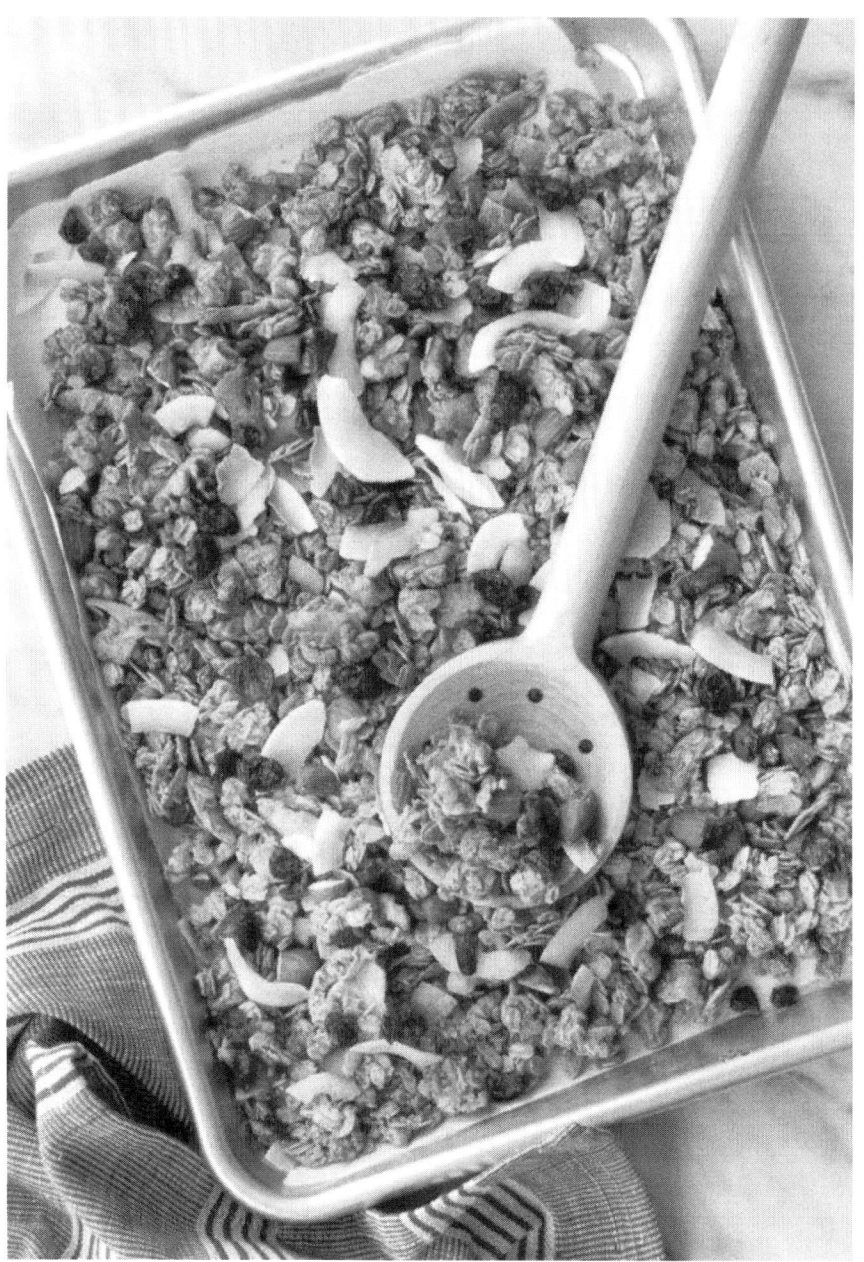

What you will need:

- 3 cups flaked oatmeal
- ¼ cup chopped raw nuts
- ¼ cup raw pecans, chopped
- ¼ cup raw almonds, chopped
- ½ cup pure maple syrup

- 2 teaspoons vanilla
- 2 teaspoons cinnamon
- 1 pinch of salt (optional)

Process:

- Preheat the oven to 250-300 ° F (149 ° C).
- Combine all ingredients in a bowl, mixing well to cover everything with maple syrup. Spread the mixture on a baking sheet or broiler pan.
- Bake until the mixture browns, stirring occasionally, 30 to 40 minutes. Transfer the baking sheet to a wire rack and let it cool completely. Keep the granola refrigerated in an airtight jar.

Nutritional values per serving:

- Calories per Zimtstern: 55 kcal
- Fat: 3.5 g
- Carbohydrates: 3.5 g
- Protein: 2 g

20. Low carb poppy seed cake

Ingredients:

- 1000 g soy quark (Alpro or Provamel)
- Something   egg substitute for three eggs
- 75 g   Nutri-plus shape & shake protein powder vanilla
- 3 tbsp semolina
- One pack custard powder (unsweetened)
- 3 tsp   liquid sweetener or sugar light (about 4-5 tbsp)
- Quantity depending on the desired intensity poppy

Preparation:

Preparation time: 20 minutes

1. Mix the egg mixture according to Preparation in a large bowl.
2. Add all remaining ingredients and stir the cream with a hand mixer.
3. Place 1/3 of the mass in a separate bowl and stir in the poppy seeds (amount depending on the desired intensity of the poppy flavor.)
4. Place the mixed layer by layer in a baking or casserole dish lined with baking paper and bake at 200 ° C (top/bottom heat) or 180 ° C (circulating air) in a preheated oven for about 60 minutes.

5. The baking or casserole dish should not exceed 20 cm in diameter. Otherwise, the cake is too flat.
6. After baking, cool (preferably in the fridge overnight) and glaze with melted dark chocolate.

Nutritional values per serving:

- Calories apiece: 112 kcal
- Carbohydrates: 3 g
- Protein: 12 g
- Fat: 6 g

21. Refreshing Blueberry Bites with Nutri-Plus Lemon Cake

Ingredients:

- 24 blueberries
- 250 g soy yogurt, unsweetened
- 20 g Nutri-plus protein powder, lemon cake

Preparation:

Preparation time: 5 minutes

You need 1-2 ice cube

1. Molds for a total of 24 yogurt bites. 1. Wash the blueberries and place each blueberry in a tray of ice cubes.
2. Stir the yogurt together with the protein powder until no more lumps are visible.
3. Carefully pour the yogurt into the ice cubes and place them in the freezer overnight.
4. Snacking is allowed at any time.

Nutritional values per serving:

- Calories per bite: 9 kcal
- Fat: 0.25 g
- Carbohydrates: 0.2 g
- Protein: 1 g

22. Chia Protein Energy Balls

Ingredients:

- 60 g ground almonds
- 60 g chopped almonds
- 60 g chia seeds

- 20 g   Nutri-plus protein powder chocolate
- 120 g Datteln

Preparation:

Preparation time: 15 minutes plus waiting time

Make 18 Energy Balls

1. Soak the dates in a little water for at least 15 minutes.
2. Add the softened dates, almonds, Chia seeds, and protein powder in a powerful blender.
3. Mix everything properly until a dough is formed.
4. Moisten your hands a little and then take about 1 tsp of dough per ball from the blender.
5. Roll the dough between your hands into small balls.
6. Optionally roll the balls in a topping of your choice. Coconut flakes, cocoa powder, chopped nuts... everything is possible.
7. Store the finished balls in the refrigerator.

Nutritional values per serving:

- Calories per ball: 81 kcal
- Fat: 5 g
- Carbohydrates: 5 g
- Protein: 3 g

23. Protein bars for the extra portion of the power

Ingredients:

- 90 g   Nutri-plus protein powder vanilla
- 30 g   coconut flower syrup
- 100 g chopped almonds
- 70 g   cashew mus
- 10 g   coconut oil
- 50ml   water
- One pinch salt
- Optional cinnamon

Preparation:

Preparation time: 15 minutes plus cooling time

Gives 400 g -> 8 bars

1. You can put all the ingredients directly into a strong blender and mix until a nice firm consistency is created.
2. Put out the mold with cling film.
3. Press the mass with your hands into the mold, and with a spoon, everything nice flat.
4. Put the mold in the fridge for at least one hour and let it set.
5. Remove the mold from the refrigerator and cut the bars into eight equal pieces.

Optional:

- ✓ Melt 30 g of dark chocolate in a water bath and gently pour over the finished bars.

Nutritional values per serving:

- Calories per bar: 190 kcal
- Fat: 12 g
- Carbohydrates: 7 g
- Protein: 14 g

24. Delicious Cinnamon Stars with Nutri-Plus Hazelnut

Ingredients:

- 150 g almonds, ground
- 200 g ground hazelnuts
- 60 g   coconut blossom sugar
- 60 g   Nutri-plus shape & shake hazelnut
- 3 tsp   cinnamon
- 5 g orange peel, abrasion
- 15 g   chia seeds
- 120 ml of   water
- 1 pinch of salt
- 100g xylitol
- 1 lemon

Preparation:

Preparation time: 45 minutes, plus cooling time

1. Stir the chia seeds into the water and let it swell slightly.
2. Put all the other ingredients, except for xylitol and lemon juice, together in a bowl and mix thoroughly.
3. Now you can add the water with the chia seeds and knead everything together.
4. Roll the dough into a ball and wrap it in cling film. Put it in the fridge for about an hour.

5. Roll the dough out about one centimeter thick and cut out little stars.
6. Repeat that until no dough is left.
7. Preheat the oven to 170 ° C and let the stars bake for about 8-10 minutes.
8. Get your stars out of the oven and let them cool.
9. Then stir the Xuckerguss from small ground xylitol and lemon juice and decorate your Zimtsterne.

Nutritional values per serving:

- Calories per Zimtstern: 55 kcal
- Fat: 3.5 g
- Carbohydrates: 3.5 g
- Protein: 2 g

25. Low carb poppy seed cake

Ingredients:

- 1000 g soy quark (Alpro or Provamel)
- Something egg substitute for 3 eggs
- 75 g   Nutri-plus shape & shake protein powder vanilla
- 3 tbsp semolina
- 1 pack custard powder (unsweetened)
- 3 tsp liquid sweetener or sugar light (about 4-5 tbsp)
- Quantity depending on the desired intensity poppy

Preparation:

Preparation time: 20 minutes

1. Mix the egg mixture according to Preparation in a large bowl.
2. Add all remaining ingredients and stir the cream with a hand mixer.
3. Place 1/3 of the mass in a separate bowl and stir in the poppy seeds (amount depending on the desired intensity of the poppy flavor.)
4. Place the mixed layer by layer in a baking or casserole dish lined with baking paper and bakc at 200 ° C (top/bottom heat) or 180 ° C (circulating air) in a preheated oven for about 60 minutes.
5. The baking or casserole dish should not exceed 20 cm in diameter; otherwise, the cake is too flat.
6. After baking, cool (preferably in the fridge overnight) and glaze with melted dark chocolate.

Nutritional values per serving:

- Calories apiece: 112 kcal
- Carbohydrates: 3 g
- Protein: 12 g
- Fat: 6 g

26. Refreshing Blueberry Bites with Nutri-Plus Lemon Cake

Ingredients:

- 24 blueberries
- 250 g soy yogurt, unsweetened
- 20 g   Nutri-plus protein powder, lemon cake

Preparation:

Preparation time: 5 minutes

You need 1-2 ice cube

1. Molds for a total of 24 yogurt bites. 1. Wash the blueberries and place each blueberry in a tray of ice cubes.
2. Stir the yogurt together with the protein powder until no more lumps are visible.
3. Carefully pour the yogurt into the ice cubes and place them in the freezer overnight.
4. Snacking is allowed at any time

Nutritional values per serving:

- Calories per bite: 9 kcal
- Fat: 0.25 g
- Carbohydrates: 0.2 g
- Protein: 1 g

27. Chia Protein Energy Balls

Ingredients:

- 60 g   ground almonds
- 60 g   chopped almonds
- 60 g   chia seeds
- 20 g   Nutri-plus protein powder chocolate
- 120 g datteln

Preparation:

Preparation time: 15 minutes plus waiting time

Make 18 Energy Balls

1. Soak the dates in a little water for at least 15 minutes.
2. Add the softened dates, almonds, Chia seeds, and protein powder in a powerful blender.
3. Mix everything properly until a dough is formed.
4. Moisten your hands a little and then take about 1 tsp of dough per ball from the blender.
5. Roll the dough between your hands into small balls.
6. Optionally roll the balls in a topping of your choice. Coconut flakes, cocoa powder, chopped nuts... everything is possible.
7. Store the finished balls in the refrigerator.

Nutritional values per serving:

- Calories per ball: 81 kcal
- Fat: 5 g
- Carbohydrates: 5 g
- Protein: 3 g

28. Protein bars for the extra portion of the power

Ingredients:

- 90 g   Nutri-plus protein powder vanilla
- 30 g   coconut flower syrup
- 100 g chopped almonds
- 70 g   cashewmus
- 10 g   coconut oil
- 50ml   water
- 1 pinch salt
- Optional cinnamon

Preparation:

Preparation time: 15 minutes plus cooling time

Gives 400 g -> 8 bars

1. You can put all the ingredients directly into a strong blender and mix until a nice firm consistency is created.
2. Put out the mold with cling film.

3. Press the mass with your hands into the mold and with a spoon, everything nice flat.
4. Put the mold in the fridge for at least one hour and let it set.
5. Remove the mold from the refrigerator and cut the bars into 8 equal pieces.

Optional:

- ✓ Melt 30 g of dark chocolate in a water bath and gently pour over the finished bars.

Nutritional values per serving:

- Calories per bar: 190 kcal
- Fat: 12 g
- Carbohydrates: 7 g
- Protein: 14 g

29. Mango Nice Cream

Ingredients:

- 2 frozen bananas
- 1 ripe mango
- 30 g Nutri-plus protein powder vanilla
- 30 ml vegetable milk
- Something mint
- Something grated chocolate

Preparation:

Preparation time: 10

1. The bananas are best frozen one day before cut into small pieces.
2. Put the bananas, the mango, the protein powder, and the soy milk together in a blender and stir until creamy.
3. Then top with mint and chocolate grated.

30. Sweet hummus dip for snacking

Ingredients:

- 480 g chickpeas (canned)
- 40 g Nutri-plus protein powder chocolate
- 30 g agave nectar
- 60 g peanut butter
- 100 ml of soy milk

- 2 teaspoons cinnamon
- 1 vanilla bean
- 1 pinch salt

Preparation:

Preparation time: 10 minutes

Results in about 600 g

1. Wash the chickpeas from the can thoroughly under running water.
2. Remove the marrow from the vanilla pod and then add all ingredients to a powerful blender.
3. Mix the mass until a homogeneous cream is produced.
4. Fill the sweet hummus in a bowl, and you can already enjoy a snack.

***TIP: Sweet or salty, you can dive pretty much anything you want. Our hummus dip is also suitable as a sweet spread or to pimp on the porridge. ***

Nutritional values per serving:

- Calories per 100 g: 170 kcal
- Fat: 6 g
- Carbohydrates: 15 g
- Protein: 13 g

31. Energy balls made from chickpeas

Ingredients:

- 90 g oatmeal
- 30 g Nutri-plus shape & shake gingerbread
- 200 g chickpeas
- 50 g dates (Medjoul)
- 20 g cocoa powder
- 1 teaspoon cinnamon
- 1 pinch salt
- 100 ml of water

Preparation:

Preparation time: 45 minutes

Make 20 Energy Ball

1. Put the oatmeal in a blender and mash to flour.

2. Wash the chickpeas very thoroughly and then add them to the blender.
3. Remove the dates and add them to the blender along with all other ingredients.
4. Let the mixer do the rest of the work and turn the mass into a solid dough.
5. Take 1 teaspoon of dough and roll it into a ball between your hands.

Optional:

- ✓ You can still roll the balls after rolling in a topping of your choice.
- ✓ Quinoa, nuts, chia seeds, cocoa powder… everything is possible.

Tip:

- ✓ The cleaner you work, the longer the balls will last longer in the fridge.
- ✓ Wear gloves best when rolling.
- ✓ It does not have to be our Shape & Shake in the taste Gingerbread!
- ✓ Vanilla, hazelnut, or chocolate are also great.

Nutritional values per serving:

- Calories per ball: 40 kcal
- Fat: 0.8 g
- Carbohydrates: 6 g
- Protein: 3 g

32. The healthy fruit bread for snacking

Ingredients:

- 100 g dried apricots
- 150 g raisins
- 125 g dried cranberries
- 2 cm ginger
- 500 ml apple juice
- 1 teaspoon lemon peels, abrasion
- 500 ml apple juice, naturally cloudy
- 100 g walnuts
- 50 g pistachios
- 50 g chopped almonds
- 50 g Nutri-plus protein powder vanilla
- 300g spelled flour
- 2 teaspoon cinnamon
- 1/2 tsp cardamom

- 1 parcel baking powder

Preparation:

Preparation time: 90 minutes, including baking time

Make a fruitcake of 1400 g

1. Cut the dried fruits into small pieces and put them together with the apple juice in a large bowl.
2. Grate the ginger, peel off the lemon zest and add both into the bowl.
3. Let it all stand for at least 30 minutes and pull through.
4. Chop the nuts roughly and mix them with the spices, the protein powder, and the baking powder.
5. Add the mixture to the dried fruit and the apple juice and mix everything.
6. Now comes the spelled flour—bit by bit. Stir the flour slowly so that no lumps form.
7. Preheat the oven to 180 ° C and layout a baking pan with baking paper.
8. Put the mass in the pan and let the bread bake for 50-60 minutes.
9. Get it out of the oven and let it cool down a bit. At best, lukewarm! If the fruit bread becomes too dark when baking, cover it with a little aluminum foil.

Nutritional values per serving:

- Calories per 100g: 280 kcal
- Fat: 9 g
- Carbohydrates: 40 g
- Protein: 9 g

33. Creamy protein chocolate with quinoa

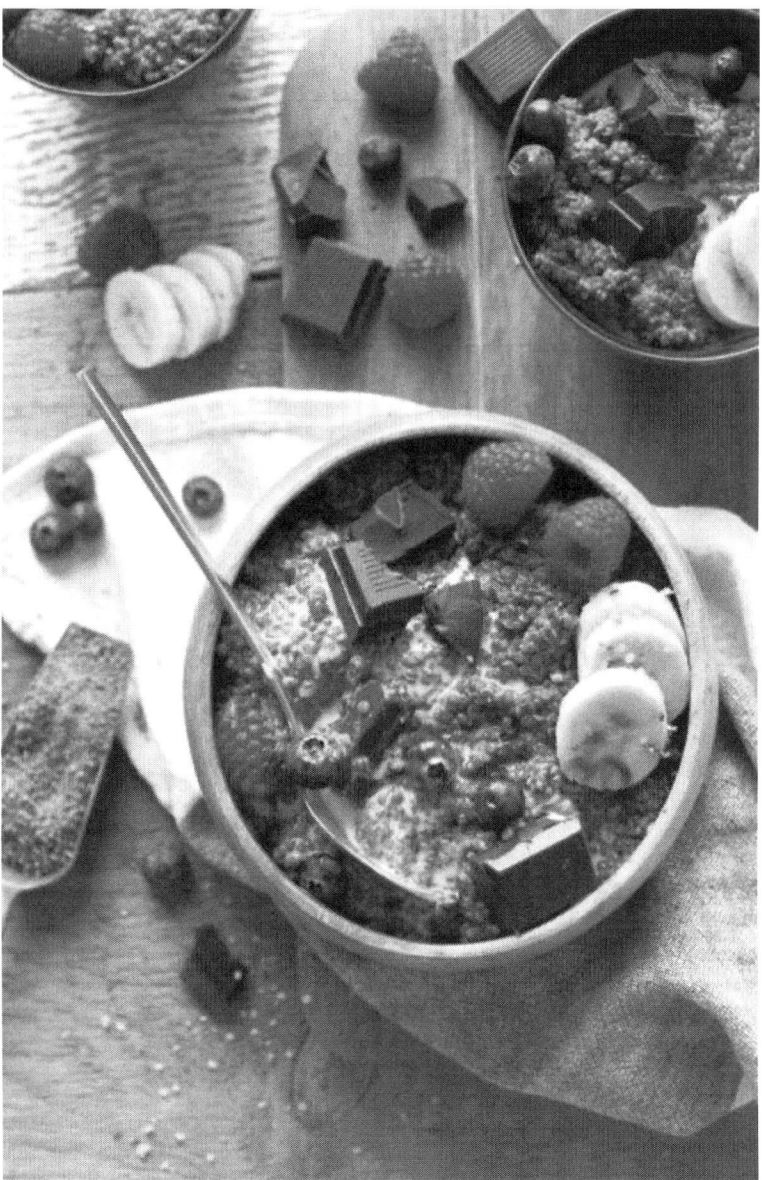

Ingredients:

- 100 g cocoa butter
- 30 g Nutri-plus protein powder chocolate
- 70 g cocoa powder
- 80 g cane sugar
- 1 vanilla bean
- 1 pinch salt
- 2 tbsp Topping of your choice, z. For example, quinoa

Preparation:

Preparation time: 1 hour, including cooling time

The amount gives a panel of about 300 g.

Of course, you can also divide the set into 2 or 3 plates.

1. Let the cocoa butter melt in a water bath.
1. Second Mix the protein powder and the cocoa powder together.
2. Add the cane sugar to the cocoa butter and stir until completely dissolved.
3. Remove everything from the heat and stir in the protein powder, cocoa mixture until no more lumps are visible.
4. Now add the marrow of a vanilla pod and stir it too.
5. Fill the liquid chocolate into a mold of your choice and add a topping. We chose quinoa and dried banana chips here.
6. Put the chocolate in the freezer for 30 minutes and then in the fridge. There it stays fresh longer, and you can treat yourself a little bit at any time.

Nutritional values per serving:

- Calories per plate: 1580 kcal
- Fat: 115 g
- Carbohydrates: 90 g
- Protein: 40 g

CHAPTER 6: VEGETABLE RECIPES

34. Boar Stew with Vegetables, Herbs and Plums, Tuscan Recipe

Ingredients:

- 1 kg wild boar from the club without fat and bone
- 1 onion
- 2 pole / s   celery
- 1 carrot
- 5 juniper berries
- 1 garlic cloves)
- 1 branch / s rosemary
- 1 branch / s marjoram or dried rubbed
- 1 branch / s thyme
- 3/ 4 liters red wine, (Chianti)
- 60 ml vinegar, (red wine vinegar)
- 3 tbsp flour
- 30 g pine nuts
- Some prune
- 30 g chocolate, bitter, grated
- 6 tbsp olive oil
- Salt
- Balsamic vinegar

Preparation:

Working time: approx. 30 min. Rest period: approx. 1 day / Level of difficulty: normal

1. Cut the wild boar meat into cubes of about the same size and place it in a bowl. Add the wine, the sliced onion, celery and carrot bits, crumbled bay leaf, crushed juniper berries, marjoram, thyme, crushed garlic, and rosemary. Cover with the marinade and let it simmer for 24 hours, stirring several times.
2. Remove the pieces of meat, drain, dab, and turn in the flour. Remove vegetables and herbs with a slotted spoon from the marinade and set aside.
3. Heat the oil in a saucepan and sauté the vegetables and herbs from the marinade. Take out and sear the meat well in the hot fat from all sides. Add the vegetables and herbs and deglaze with the marinade. Cover and stew for about 3 hours on the lowest heat setting.

4. After 1 ½ hours, remove the meat with a slotted spoon and place on a plate. Fish the herb sprigs from the sauce and purée the gravy carefully with a wand. Put the meat and sauce back in the pot. Add the finely chopped pine nuts, the prunes, cut into fine strips, and the dark chocolate. Pour in the red wine vinegar and stew for another 1 ½ hours. Season with some balsamic vinegar and salt.

Nutrition Facts:

Serving Size: 1 serving Amount Per Serving

- Calories: 247.2
- Protein: 7.5 g
- Vitamin A: 110.5 %
- Iron: 11.2 %
- Zinc: 7.5 %

35. Turkish Acma With Sheep's Cheese and Vegetables

Ingredients:

For the dough:

- 100 ml water
- 100 ml milk
- 100 ml oil
- 200 g quark
- 1 tbsp salt
- 3 tbsp sugar
- 2 pck. yeast, fresh
- 100 ml cream
- 700 g Flour
- 1 pck. baking powder for the filling:
- 200 g feta cheese
- 1 / 2 bund parsley

For the decoration:

- 10 cherry tomato
- 2 pepperonis
- 10 olives
- 1 egg yolk

Preparation:

Working time: approx. 40 min.

Cooking/baking time: approx. 25 min. Rest period: approx. 1 hr.

Difficulty level: simple

1. For the dough, mix all the liquid ingredients. Mix the flour and baking powder, add gradually and prepare the dough. Leave the dough in a warm place for 45 minutes.
2. Form small balls from the dough, brushing the hands with oil. Lay out a baking tray with baking paper and place the balls over it. Cover your hands with oil now and then. Make a recess with your fingers into the balls and fill them with sheep's cheese and parsley. Decorate with tomatoes, peppers, and olives, and let the balls go for another 15 minutes.
3. Brush with egg yolks and bake in a preheated oven at 160 ° C for 20 - 25 minutes.

Nutrition Facts:

Serving Size: 1 serving Amount Per Serving

- Calories: 88.0 kcal
- Saturated Fat: 0.2 g
- Cholesterol: 13.4 mg
- Sodium: 107.1 mg
- Protein: 7.9 g
- Vitamin A: 38.9 %

36. My creamy, vegan peanut fritters with vegetables and soy

Vegan recipe (of course vegetarian) 2 portions

Ingredients:

- 3 / 4 cup   soya granules
- Vegetable broth, hot, for soaking
- 1 m. large Onion (s), diced
- 1 garlic clove (s), crushed
- 1 / 2 m.-large carrot (s), diced
- 1 / 2 m.-large zucchini, diced
- 1 can corn, (or 140g vegetable corn)
- 100 ml vegetable stock, strong
- 150 ml soy milk (soy drink)
- 3 tbsp soy sauce

- 3 tbsp peanut butter
- 1 tbsp parsley
- something chili powder
- something pepper
- Possibly. curry powder
- Possibly. paprika
- something vegetable oil, for searing
- Possibly. flour, to thicken

Preparation:

Working time: approx. 30 min.

Cooking/baking time: approx. 20 min. Rest period: approx. 5 min.

Difficulty level: simple

1. Soy granules in a bowl. Bring the vegetable stock to a boil and pour over the granules. It should not be in the "dry" and swell well. Let it swell for at least 5 minutes. Then express properly and possibly season with a little salt or broth (can taste nice strong).
2. Heat vegetable oil in the pan and add the granules. The best taste is achieved in my opinion, if you let the granules neatly burn until it is nicely browned and crispy.
3. Then add the diced onions, carrots, and the crushed garlic clove and also lightly brown.
4. Finally, add the diced zucchini and corn.
5. Add the mixture of soymilk, vigorous vegetable broth, and soy sauce.
6. The peanut butter (I like it very creamy and add 4 tablespoons), add pepper and chili powder.
7. Cover and simmer everything until the zucchini are done. If it has become too thick, add some soy milk or water. Finally, to taste again.
8. The sauce should be nice creamy with a good spiciness and seasoning. If necessary, add a little broth, salt, chili powder, or pepper. If you like it even thicker, you can of course also thicken with some flour. Also, there is rice for me. If you like, you can also choose the other side dishes.
9. Some fresh parsley provides the last whistle.

Nutrition Facts:

Serving Size: 1 serving Amount Per Serving

- Calories: 281.5 kcal
- Protein: 13.8 g
- Vitamin A: 0.7 %
- Vitamin C: 5.2 %

37. Bolognese Sauce with Lots of Vegetables

1 portion

Ingredients:

- 2 tbsp oil
- 1 kg minced meat, from beef
- 500 g soup vegetables, (carrot, leek, celery)
- 1 carrot
- 2 onion
- 2 garlic cloves
- 1 small one hot peppers, hot
- 50 ml red wine, dry
- 800 g tomato (s), from the tin, pieced with juice
- 3 tsp oregano, dried
- 1 / 2 tsp basil, dried
- 1 bay leaf
- 1 pinch sugar
- 250 ml beef broth, seasoned
- 2 Teaspoons
- Salt, approx.
- 1 / 4 TL black pepper
- 1 teaspoon beef broth, instant, approx.

Preparation:

Working time: approx. 35 min.

Cooking time: approx. 4 hrs. 20 min.

Level of difficulty: normal

1. First, in a separate pan, mince the minced meat in the hot oil until it is crumbly. That takes about 10 minutes. Drain the fat as best as possible, but leave about 3 tablespoons in the pan. Put the minced meat in the ceramic pot. Now clean the vegetables - carrots, onions, leeks, celery, garlic, and hot peppers - as usual, and, if possible, grate them roughly in a food processor. The vegetable mixture is then gently cooked in the remaining oil over medium heat. Deglaze with a good red wine (but do not boil) and give everything to the minced meat. Finally, add the spices, the dried herbs, and the liquids. Carefully mix and level slightly. Do not be

alarmed, the Bolognese seems very plump - but that's the way it should be! The Schmorzeit is approx. 2 hours HIGH and 2 - 3 hours LOW.

2. In between, you may also stir. Season with salt, pepper, and a little more brewing powder.
3. Serve with spaghetti and sprinkle with grated hard cheese (eg Parmesan).

Nutrition Facts:

Serving Size: 1 serving Amount Per Serving

- Calories: 271.2 kcal
- Protein: 10.1 g
- Vitamin A: 42.7 %
- Vitamin C: 14.8 %

38. Vegetables - Lasagna A La Mousse

6 portions

Ingredients:

- Lasagne plate (s) (without egg - without precooking)
- 1 big one   onion (s), finely diced
- 2 toe / n garlic, finely chopped
- 2 m. -Large Zucchini, grated
- 2 m. -Large Carrot (s), grated
- 1 m. -Large Pepper (s), red, small diced
- 2 pole / s   celery, in fine slices
- 200 g mushrooms, in fine slices
- 400 g sour cream
- 150 g cheese, raw milk Emmentaler, grated
- 1 tbsp olive oil
- salt and pepper
- chili powder
- 400 g Herbal cream cheese or light herb cream cheese
- 2 toe garlic, crushed
- something water
- 100 g parmesan, grated
- Olive oil, for the form

Preparation:

Working time: approx. 45 min. Rest period: approx. 5 hrs. / Difficulty level: normal

1. Heat the olive oil in a large, coated pan (or wok) and fry the onion, garlic and vegetables vigorously for 5 minutes. Remove the pan/wok from the griddle and cool briefly and mix in the sour cream and cheese.
2. Mix the herb cream cheese with the garlic and enough water to make a very creamy sauce.
3. Rub a large casserole dish well with olive oil.
4. First, so much cream cheese sauce that the casserole is well covered, then "stratified": a layer of lasagne leaves, cream cheese sauce, a layer of vegetables, a layer of lasagne leaves, cream cheese sauce, vegetables, etc. The last two layers should be lasagna leaves and cream cheese Be sauce.
5. Cover the lasagne with aluminum foil or a lid and leave to soak in the refrigerator for at least 5 hours (better longer, up to 12 hours).
6. Preheat the oven to 180 degrees top/bottom heat.
7. Sprinkle the grated Parmesan cheese over the lasagna and bake for 45 minutes.

39. Fried Noodles with Vegetables and Meat (Asian)

2 portions

Ingredients:

- 200 g Chinese egg noodles
- 2 liters water
- 1 tbsp salt
- 2 tbsp oil
- 200 g pork or turkey meat
- 3 spring onions
- 1 pepper
- 2 carrot
- Some broccolis
- 1 / 4 liters Water, hot
- 1 teaspoon broth, grained
- 2 tbsp soy sauce
- 1 tbsp corn-starch
- Salt and pepper
- 2 tbsp oil
- Soy sauce

Preparation:

Working time: approx. 20 min.

Difficulty level: normal

1. Boil the noodles in the boiling salted water according to the packing instructions and strain.
2. Fry the meat in a large pan with oil for 3 minutes.
3. Clean the spring onions, wash and cut into 2 cm long pieces. Wash the peppers, cut in half, corer them and cut into strips. Wash the carrots, peel and grate or cut into thin slices. And wash the broccoli.
4. Add the sliced vegetables to the meat in the pan and fry for 2 minutes.
5. Mix the stock, soy sauce, and corn-starch well in a bowl, add to the frying pan and add to the ingredients.
6. Heat the oil in another pan, add the drained noodles and cook for about 3 minutes. Then add the vegetable-meat mixture and mix.
7. Put in a preheated bowl.

Nutrition Facts:

Serving Size: 1 serving

- Calories: 190.0 kcal
- Total Fat: 7.0 g
- Saturated Fat: 0.0 g
- Cholesterol: 0.0 mg
- Sodium: 0.0 mg
- Potassium: 0.0 mg
- Total Carbohydrates: 22.0 g
- Dietary Fiber: 1.0 g
- Sugar: 1.0 g
- Protein: 10.0 g

40. Salmon with Vegetables and Potatoes

3 portions

Ingredients:

- 1 salmon (wild salmon, in whole)
- 6 m. -Large Potato
- 4 m. -Large Carrot
- 2 broccolis
- 4 m. -Large Tomatoes
- 1 / 4 liters vegetable stock

- 1 cup cream
- 2 tbsp herbs, French (or of your choice), chopped
- Butter, cut into flakes
- Salt and pepper

Preparation:

Working time: approx. 30 min.

Cooking/baking time: approx. 30 min.

Level of difficulty: normal

1. Peel the potatoes and carrots. Divide the broccoli into florets. Halve the potatoes and cut the carrots into 3 - 5 cm long pieces.
2. Cook the potatoes and carrots for about 10 minutes and the broccoli in salted water for about 3 minutes. Drain the water and distribute the potatoes and vegetables on the meat pan from the oven. Divide the salmon into about eight portions and place between vegetables and potatoes. Wash the tomatoes, cut crosswise, and also put on the tin. Now mix the broth and cream with the herbs, salt, and pepper (Tip: If you love garlic, you can also add it to the broth). Now pour this broth over the ingredients on the plate and spread butter flakes over the vegetables and salmon as needed.
3. Cook in the preheated oven at 200 ° C circulating air for approx. 30 minutes. Serve hot.
4. The recipe can also be prepared well for a party and - when it's time - simply put it in the oven.

Nutrition Facts:

Serving Size: 1 serving Amount Per Serving

- Calories: 337.9 kcal
- Total Fat: 16.5 g
- Saturated Fat: 2.5 g
- Cholesterol: 80.5 mg
- Sodium: 97.0 mg
- Potassium: 1,242.6 mg
- Total Carbohydrates: 15.7 g
- Dietary Fiber: 3.0 g
- Sugar: 3.3 g
- Protein: 31.6 g

41. Fried Salmon on Mediterranean Vegetables

2 portions

Ingredients:

- 4 Pepper (s), red, coarsely crushed
- 1 m. -Large Eggplant (s), roughly minced
- 1m. -Large Zucchini, roughly minced
- 1 bunch vegetable onion (s), roughly chopped
- 750 g salmon fillet (s) (TK), thawed, pieced
- 1 Lemon (s), the juice of it
- 1 glass pesto (basil pesto)
- Flour
- Seasoned salt
- Olive oil
- Vegetable stock
- Ketchup (curry ketchup), spicy
- Paprika
- Pepper
- 1 pinch sugar
- Fat for the mold

Preparation:

Working time: approx. 35 min.

Difficulty level: normal

1. Fry the prepared vegetables in a large pan while stirring with the hot olive oil. Add a little vegetable stock and let it simmer for about 7-10 minutes with the lid. Season with curry ketchup, herbal salt, paprika, pepper, and sugar as needed.
2. In the meantime, marinate the thawed salmon pieces with lemon juice and then season with herb salt. Turn in a little flour and brown on both sides in olive oil.
3. Put the vegetables in a greased casserole dish, arrange the salmon pieces on top, and spread generously with the basil pesto.
4. In the preheated oven overcool at 200 ° C convection for about 7-10 minutes.
5. This tastes like a baguette or flatbread.

Nutrition Facts:

Serving Size: 1 serving Amount Per Serving

- Calories: 113.4 kcal
- Total Fat: 5.4 g
- Saturated Fat: 0.8 g
- Cholesterol: 0.0 mg
- Sodium: 539.2 mg
- Potassium: 464.4 mg
- Total Carbohydrates: 16.3 g
- Dietary Fiber: 4.8 g
- Sugars: 5.6 g
- Protein: 2.7 g

42. Oven Chicken with Vegetables

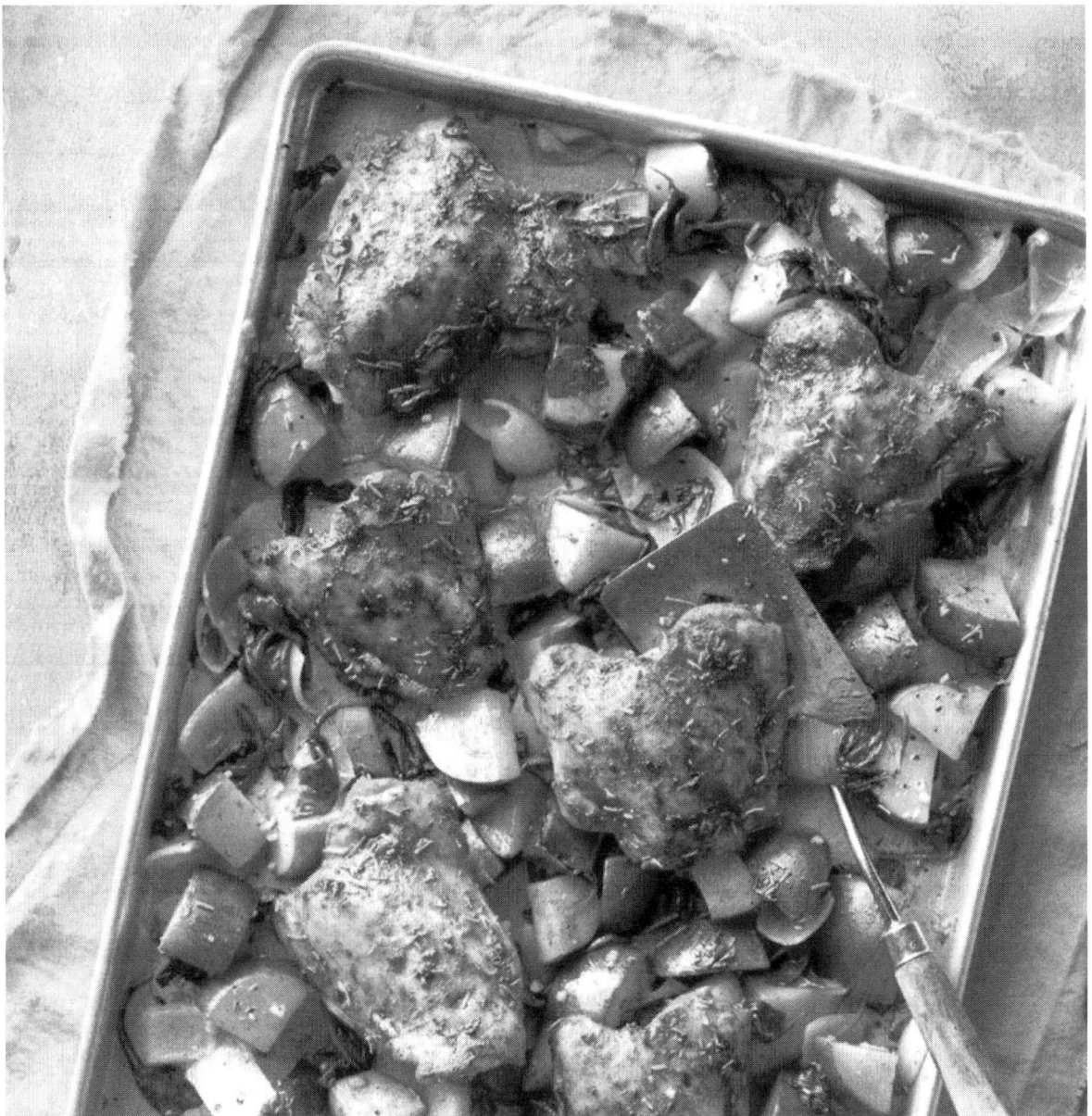

4 portions

Ingredients:

- Chicken legs, fresh or frozen
- Potato
- Carrot
- Toe garlic, roughly chopped
- Onion
- 100 ml olive oil
- 1 teaspoon paprika powder, sweet

- 1 teaspoon paprika powder, pink
- 1 teaspoon salt
- 1 teaspoon thyme
- Toe garlic, pressed

Preparation:

Working time: approx. 30 min.

Cooking/baking time: approx. 1 hr.

Difficulty level: simple

1. Peel and dice the potatoes and carrots. Peel and halve the onion, finely dice one half and cut the other into rings. Add together with 2 coarsely chopped garlic cloves to the potato and carrot cubes.
2. Then mix a marinade with oil, paprika, salt, thyme, and pressed garlic. So that the chicken thighs brush (very important: also marinade under the skin!). Add the rest of the marinade to 1 - 2 teaspoons of the potato and carrot mixture and mix well, season with salt, if necessary.
3. Put the vegetable mixture into a large baking dish, put the chicken thighs on top, and bake at 200 ° C for 60 - 70 minutes. Possibly. brush with remaining marinade. After about half of the baking time, I turn the thighs and let them take some color from below for a few minutes. To make the skin crispy, but in any case, turn it again a few minutes before the end of cooking time.
4. Vegetables and meat become very fragrant when they are baked together and after the schnippelei the whole thing cooks itself by itself. With certainty, the recipe can also be changed with other vegetables (zucchini, paprika, ...) or other spices.

Nutrition Facts:

Serving Size: 1 serving Amount Per Serving

- Calories: 328.6 kcal
- Total Fat: 8.8 g
- Saturated Fat: 1.4 g
- Cholesterol: 68.4 mg
- Sodium: 181.8 mg
- Potassium: 1,174.8 mg
- Total Carbohydrates: 30.6 g
- Dietary Fiber: 4.1 g
- Sugar: 1.5 g
- Protein: 30.9

43. Beef Steak with Mustard and Herb Topping and Vegetables

4 portions

Ingredients:

- Thick beef steak (s) (beef steaks), each about 250 g, well-hung
- Large carrot
- m. -Large zucchini
- 2 TL, heaped mustard medium hot
- something herbs of Provence
- something pepper
- something salt (Society Garlic salt) or Himalayan salt
- something olive oil or coconut oil
- Herbs, fresh (thyme, garlic, mushroom)
- something Leeks or onions, optional

Preparation:

Working time: approx. 10 min.

Cooking/baking time: approx. 6 min. Rest period: approx. 3 hrs. 10 min.

Level of difficulty: normal

1. Rub the two steaks well with olive oil and cover for at least 3 hours in the fridge (better already 1 day before). Half an hour before frying (preferably in an iron pan) take out of the refrigerator. Preheat the oven to 80 ° C without circulating air.
2. Make the pan very hot and fry the steaks without further oil. Fry for
3. - 2 (otherwise 3) minutes on each side, depending on the thickness.
4. Sprinkle the steaks with mustard, sprinkle with Provence pepper and herbs, wrap in aluminum foil, and place in the oven. Let rest for 10-15 minutes. The steaks are salted after resting.
5. In the meantime, peel the carrots, wash the zucchini, and cut both into small pieces. Fry in a pan with 2 tablespoons of coconut oil (if necessary, sauté onions and leeks) and let it cook. Season with salt, pepper, and fresh herbs to taste.

44. Protein Cream Biscuits

5 people

Prep: 15 mins

Ingredients:

- 1 egg
- 60 g oatmeal, ground or instant oats from foodspring
- 1 pinch salt
- Optional some chocolate droplets, bittersweet

Make biscuits yourself with only 3 ingredients. Sounds as easy as it is. If you are a big fan of our protein cream, you are also a fan of this recipe!

Preparation:

1. We baked 5 cookies from the mass. 1 biscuit has about 176 kcal and 7 g of protein.
2. Preheat the oven to 160 degrees.
3. Put all ingredients in a bowl. Mix until a homogeneous mass is obtained.
4. Add the chocolate droplets as desired.
5. Remove 1 tbsp each, form a ball, flatten and place on a baking tray lined with baking paper.

Tip: You get 5-6 biscuits from the dough. Bake in the oven for 10 minutes.

Nutrition Facts per Serving:

- Calories: 176 kcal - 383 kcal / 100 g
- Carbohydrates: 16 g - 34 g / 100 g
- Proteins: 7 g - 16 g / 100 g
- Fat: 10 g - 22 g / 100 g

45. Protein Cream Biscuits Chocolate Cookies From A Few Ingredients

1 person

Prep: 15 mins

Ingredients:

- 1 egg
- 60 g oatmeal, ground or instant oats from foodspring
- 1 pinch salt
- Optional some chocolate droplets, bittersweet

Make biscuits yourself with only 3 ingredients. Sounds as easy as it is. If you are a big fan of our protein cream, you are also a fan of this recipe!

Preparation:

1. We baked 5 cookies from the mass. 1 biscuit has about 176 kcal and 7g of protein.
2. Preheat the oven to 160 degrees.
3. Put all ingredients in a bowl. Mix until a homogeneous mass is obtained.
4. Add the chocolate droplets as desired.
5. Remove 1 tbsp each, form a ball, flatten and place on a baking tray lined with baking paper.

*** Tip: You get 5-6 biscuits from the dough. Bake in the oven for 10 minutes.***

Nutrition Facts per Serving:

- Calories: 176 kcal - 383 kcal / 100 g
- Carbohydrates: 16 g - 34 g / 100 g
- Proteins: 7 g - 16 g / 100 g
- Fat: 10 g - 22 g / 100 g

46. Vegan Protein Pancakes Fluffy Pancakes Without Eggs

1 person

Ingredients:

- 90 g oatmeal, ground or instant oats from foodspring
- 30 g
- 1 tsp baking powder
- 1 pinch salt
- 230 ml sparkling water

Optional Toppings: blueberries, maple syrup, etc.

You do not need much for your delicious, vegan Sunday breakfast. From your protein powder, which you have only used for shakes, you can conjure fluffy protein pancakes. Convince yourself!

Preparation:

1. From the dough, we baked 4 pancakes. The whole portion has 453 kcal and 31 g of protein.
2. Mix all dry ingredients in a bowl.
3. Add the water slowly and stir with a whisk until a thick dough is formed.
4. Heat a pan with a little oil and bake the pancakes in it.
5. Serve with toppings at will.

Nutrition Facts per Serving:

- Calories: 453 kcal - 128 kcal / 100 g
- Carbohydrates: 66 g - 19 g / 100 g

- Proteins: 31 g - 9 g / 100 g
- Fat: 7 g - 2 g / 100 g

47. Vegan Brownies Recipe Juicy, Chocolaty, Sugar-Free

1 person

Ingredients:

- Bananas, very ripe
- 90 g apple purée, unsweetened
- 30 g oatmeal, ground or instant oats from foodspring
- 40 g cocoa powder, unsweetened
- 1 pinch salt
- 60 ml oat milk
- Optional 25 g of chocolate droplets, bittersweet

Our vegans are finally getting their money's worth! We show how to bake delicious protein brownies without animal ingredients. And without sugar. But all the more chocolaty and juicy!

Preparation:

1. If you cut the brownies into 6 pieces, 1 piece has about 110 kcal and 6 g of protein.
2. Preheat oven to 175 degrees.
3. Crush the bananas in a bowl with a fork. Mix with the applesauce.
4. Add the oatmeal, cocoa powder, protein powder, and salt and mix everything. Add the milk until a dough is formed.
5. Put the dough in an angular, greased shape. Sprinkle chocolate over it at will.
6. Bake in the oven for 25-30 minutes. Allow to cool before consumption.

Nutrition Facts per Serving:

- Calories: 110 kcal - 134 Kcal / 100 g
- Carbohydrates: 15 g - 18 g / 100 g
- Proteins: 6 g - 7 g / 100 g
- Fat: 2 g - 3 g / 100 g

48. Protein Chia Pudding with Irresistible Chocolate Candy

1 person

Ingredients:

For the pudding:

- 200 ml milk (1.5% Fat)
- 15 g shape shake at the option of foodspring

For the topping:

- 50 g raspberries, fresh or frozen
- g brazil nuts, chopped

Since the launch of our heavenly protein cream, we will beat pretty much any sweet treat with it. Like this Chia Pudding. With a decent amount of protein, it is the perfect breakfast for you and your muscles.

Preparation:

1. The recipe results in a pudding with 454 Kcal and 29 g of protein.
2. Mix all ingredients for the pudding. This works well with your shaker, for example.
3. Let it soak in the fridge for at least 30 minutes or overnight.
4. In a bowl and fill with toppings serve.

Nutrition Facts per Serving:

- Calories: 454 kcal - 142 kcal / 100 g
- Carbohydrates: 20 g - 6 g / 100 g
- Proteins: 29 g - 9 g / 100 g
- Fat: 26 g - 8 g / 100 g

49. Oatmeal Seasoned with Vegetables

What you will need:

- 4 cups of water
- 2 cups of "cut" oatmeal (quick-cooking steel-cut oats)
- 1 teaspoon Italian spices
- ½ teaspoon "herbamare" or sea salt
- 1 teaspoon garlic powder
- 1 teaspoon onion powder
- ½ cup nutritional yeast
- ¼ teaspoon turmeric powder
- 1½ cup kale or tender spinach
- ½ cup sliced mushrooms
- ¼ cup grated carrots
- ½ cup small chopped peppers

Process:

1. Boil the water in a saucepan.
2. Add the oatmeal and spices and lower the temperature.
3. Cook over low heat without lid for 5 to 7 minutes.
4. Add the vegetables.
5. Cover and set aside for 2 minutes.
6. Serve immediately.

50. Crushed Olives Paste

What you will need:

- 2 cups unprocessed whole grain pasta (I like Jovial [optional: quinoa])
- 20 or more crushed, chopped, and chopped olives
- 4 cloves garlic, minced
- 1 bunch of parsley with stems, all chopped
- 1 tablespoon red chili flakes (less than that if you don't like spicy)
- Water to heat olives, garlic, and parsley (optional: oil)
- Salt and pepper, if you wish
- Green leafy vegetable of your choice (I love arugula)

Process:

1. Boil the water in a large pot, add the pasta, stirring occasionally.
2. Wash the parsley, arugula (or another green leafy vegetable of your choice)
3. Crush the garlic and chop the parsley.
4. Crush the olives, remove the seeds and chop them lightly.
5. When the pasta is cooked, drain it and set it aside.
6. Heat the pan, add a little water and add 1 tablespoon (or less) of red pepper flakes, chopped parsley, garlic, and olives. Fry them for about 2 to 3 minutes, making sure you keep stirring this mixture — don't let the garlic burn.
7. Add the cooked pasta and mix.
8. Turn off the heat.
9. Add the arugula and mix (the arugula will wilt or cook slightly by the heat of the pasta).

CHAPTER 7: SMOOTHIES AND JUICES

51. Carrot Drink with Parsley and Lemon with Garlic

Ingredients:

For 2 portions:

- 2 small cloves of garlic
- 800 g bunch of carrots
- 1 bunch smooth parsley
- ½ lemon
- 1 tsp rapeseed oil

Preparation:

1. Peel garlic cloves.
2. Thoroughly wash carrots and cut off the ends.
3. Wash parsley and shake dry. Squeeze lemon half off.
4. Juice garlic and 6 carrots in the juicer.
5. Add parsley and remaining carrots to the juicer and juice.
6. Mix carrot drink with about 2 tablespoons of lemon juice and the rapeseed oil and enjoy immediately.

52. Spicy tomato-thick milk drink

Ingredients:

For 2 portions:

- ½ red chili pepper
- 3 stems basil
- 275 g junket
- 1 tsp olive oil
- Salt
- Pepper
- ½ lemon
- 200 ml tomato juice

Preparation:

1. Rinse half chili pepper, dry, remove seeds and finely chop. Wash the basil, shake dry, peel off the leaves, cover some with garnish if necessary, finely chop the others.

2. Mix the chili and basil with the thick milk and olive oil, season with salt and pepper. Fill in 2 glasses and refrigerate for about 15 minutes.
3. Squeeze out the lemon. Tomato juice with about 1 tablespoon of lemon juice, salt, and pepper to taste spicy.
4. Carefully pour the tomato juice into the glasses with the thick milk, so that 2 layers are formed, eg run over a spoon back into the glass. Garnish with basil and serve immediately.

53. Apple Cherry Cocktail with Celery

Ingredients:

For 1 serving:

- 1 red apple (about 200 g)
- 2 bars celery (about 100 g each)
- 200 g sour cherries (pitted, frozen)

Preparation:

1. Wash, dry, halve, and dice the apple.
2. Wash the celery stalks, clean them, remove them if necessary and cut into pieces.
3. Wash the celery green and shake dry.
4. Juice the apple and celery with about 2/3 of the celery green juice in a juicer.
5. Add chilled cherries to the juice and puree with a hand blender. Pour into a glass and garnish with the remaining celery green.

54. Apple Vegetable Juice with Beetroot

Ingredients:

For 2 portions:

- 3 carrots (à 100 g)
- 2 apples (à 200 g)
- 2 tubers rote bete (à 125 g)
- ½ lemon
- 1 tl rapeseed oil

Preparation:

1. Carrot thoroughly and cut small. Wash apples, quarter, and possibly core.
2. Thoroughly wash the beetroot, peel it with a peeler at will or roughly chop it with the peel, possibly working with gloves because of the color.
3. Juice carrots, apples, and beets with a mechanical juicer.

4. Squeeze out the lemon and measure 2 tablespoons of juice. Stir with the rapeseed oil under the apple and vegetable juice and serve immediately.

55. Strong vegetable juice with ginger

Ingredients:

For 2 portions:

- 1 cucumber
- 1 big beetroot
- 5 bars celery
- 2 carrots
- 1 piece of ginger root (about 25 g)
- 1 tsp argan oil

Preparation:

1. Wash the cucumber and quarter it.
2. Wash, clean, and quarter beetroot.
3. Wash, clean, and remove celery. Wash carrots and cut off the ends.
4. Wash ginger and cut into pieces.
5. Process vegetables in the juicer, mix with argan oil, and drink immediately.

56. Fast Beetroot Drink with Chives

Ingredients:

For 1 portion:

- 1 onion (about 50 g)
- 1 clove of garlic
- 150 ml beetroot juice
- 50 ml carrot juice
- 3 stalks of chives
- also: ice cubes

Preparation:

1. Peel onion and garlic. Cut the onion into pieces and squeeze over a glass with a garlic press.
2. Press garlic, stir in beetroot and carrot juice well. Add ice cubes. Wash the chives, shake dry and garnish with the drink.

57. Paprika Cocktail with orange

Ingredients:

For 1 serving:

- 1 stalk mint
- 1 green pepper (about 200 g)
- 1 yellow pepper (about 200 g)
- 2 juicy oranges (à 125 g)
- also: ice cubes

Preparation:

1. Wash mint, shake dry, and peel off the leaves. Halve, corer, wash and quarter bell peppers.
2. Cut the oranges in half and squeeze them out.
3. Finely chop ice cubes in an ice crusher and pour it into a glass. Juice the pieces of pepper in a juicer and stir in the glass with the orange juice. Garnish with mint.

58. Red Apple Juice with Red Cabbage

Ingredients:

For 1 portion:

- 2 sweet red apples
- 1-piece red cabbage (200 g)
- 1 tsp balsamic vinegar
- Ice cubes

Preparation:

1. Wash, dry, and quarter the apples.
2. Clean red cabbage, wash it and chop it roughly. Cut a small piece for the garnish into narrow strips.
3. Juicing apples and red cabbage in a juicer. Stir in a glass with balsamic vinegar and ice cubes. Garnish with the red cabbage strips and enjoy immediately.

59. Spicy Carrot Juice with Curry Foam

Ingredients:

For 1 portion:

- ½ small lime

- 1 stalk coriander
- ½ tl mild curry powder
- ½ tl hot curry powder
- 150 ml carrot juice
- 30 ml milk (1.5%, preferably h-milk)

Preparation:

1. Squeeze out half of the lime.
2. Wash cilantro, shake dry, peel off leaves, and cut into thin strips.
3. Mixing mild and spicy curry powder in a small bowl.
4. Put the carrot juice and lime juice with 2/3 of the curry mixture in a tall container and mix briefly with a hand blender.
5. Stir the remaining curry mixture with the milk and use a milk frother to make a fine-pored, stiff foam. Put the carrot juice in a tall glass, put the curry foam on it with a spoon, sprinkle with coriander and enjoy.

60. Cucumber-orange drink

Ingredients:

For 4 glasses:

- ½ Cucumber
- 1 bunch mint
- ½ lime juice
- 3 oranges

Preparation:

1. Wash the half of the cucumber, halve lengthwise, corer and dice.
2. Wash mint, shake dry, and peel off leaves.
3. Puree the cucumber and mint in a blender.
4. Squeeze lime half and oranges and mix with the cucumber puree.

61. Cucumber drink with wasabi

Ingredients:

For 1 portion (125 ml):

- 4 stems dill
- 1-piece cucumber (100 g)
- Sea-salt

- 1 tsp wasabi
- White pepper
- 50 ml milk (1.5% fat) (cold)

Preparation:

1. Wash dill, shake dry, and finely chop. Wash the cucumber and pat dry.
2. Cut a bite-sized piece from the cucumber and cut it lengthwise with two closely spaced cuts to 2/3 of the length. Lightly fan and stick on a wooden skewer.
3. Peel the remaining cucumber, dice, and finely puree with dill and a little salt. Then pass the cucumber mixture through a sieve lined with a cloth.
4. Mix the collected cucumber liquid with wasabi paste, pepper, and milk, season to taste with salt, and pour into a glass. Serve garnished with the cucumber skewer.

62. Cucumber Smoothie

Ingredients:

For 2 portions:

- 1-piece cucumber about 200 g
- 1 shallot
- 1 tbsp chopped dill tips
- 150 g yogurt
- 70 ml cold milk
- Salt
- Black pepper
- Tabasco
- 2 splashes Worcester sauce
- Mint leaf around garnish

Preparation:

1. Wash cucumber, peel, and chop. Peel the shallot, chop and add to the blender with cucumber, dill, yogurt, and milk and finely puree. Season with salt, pepper, Tabasco, and Worcester's sauce and mix everything briefly.
2. To serve, pour into two glasses and garnish with mint leaves.

63. Cucumber smoothie with muesli

Ingredients:

For 4 portions:

- For the cereal
- 150 g oatmeal
- 100 g hazelnuts
- 4 tbsp liquid honey
- 8th strawberries
- 50 g raspberries
- 500 g yogurt
- For the shake
- Cayenne pepper

Preparation:

1. Wash the cucumber, cut off the ends, peel, and dice. Freeze in the freezer for about 30 minutes.
2. Rinse the dill, clean it, spin it dry and chop it roughly. Puree with the cucumber, the yogurt, a little buttermilk, and the lemon juice in a blender. Add the remaining buttermilk and puree until the shake is creamy. Season with salt and cayenne pepper and fill into 4 small bottles at will.
3. For the cereal, mix the oatmeal with the nuts mixed into cups. Drizzle the honey over it. Wash, clean, and cut the strawberries. Read the raspberries and spread them together with the strawberries on the cereals. Add the yogurt and serve with the shake.

64. Cucumber and Blackberry Smoothie

Ingredients:

For 4 glasses (150 ml):

- 200 g fresh ripe blackberry
- ½ cucumber
- 400 ml apple juice
- 1 el lemon juice
- Sugar to taste

Preparation:

1. Wash the blackberries and drain. Peel the cucumber, cut it in half, corer it, cut it into small cubes, and finely puree it with the blackberries and the apple juice in a blender.
2. Season with lemon juice and sugar and serve well chilled in glasses.

65. Spicy carrot drink

Ingredients:

For 2 portions:

- 3 big carrots
- 2 brazil nuts
- 50 ml low-fat milk
- 100 ml tomato juice
- 2 splashes tabasco
- Salt
- Pepper
- 1 sprig of thyme

Preparation:

1. Wash carrots and juice one half. Chop Brazil nuts and stir. Add milk and tomato juice and stir well.
2. Season with Tabasco, salt, and pepper until spicy. Remove some thyme leaves from the stalk and stir in the juice mixture.
3. Fill the carrot and milk mixture into a tall glass and decorate with the remaining carrot half and the sprigs of thyme.

66. Green Smoothies with Yogurt

Ingredients:

For 4 portions:

- 200 g green asparagus
- Salt
- 80 g peas
- 1 banana
- 1 tbsp lemon juice
- 1 little apple
- 100 g baby spinach
- 1 handful
- Apple mint (hain mint)
- 400 g yogurt
- 100 ml mineral water or apple juice
- 1 pinch

- Sugar
- 2 radishes

Preparation:

1. Peel the asparagus in the lower third and cut off woody ends. Cook in boiling salted water with the peas for about 8 minutes. Then drain, chill off ice-cold and drain. Cut the asparagus tips about 8 cm long and set aside for the garnish.
2. Peel the banana and cut into pieces. Mix with the lemon juice. Peel the apple, cut it to size and mix with the banana. Wash the spinach thoroughly. Rinse the mint and pluck the leaves. Add together with the fruit, vegetables, and yogurt in the blender and finely puree. If necessary, add a little water or juice to the desired consistency. Season with a pinch of sugar and salt.
3. Clean the radishes, wash and cut into thin slices. Halve the asparagus tips lengthwise. Spread the smoothie on glasses and serve garnished with the radishes and asparagus.

CHAPTER 8: DESSERT RECIPES

67. Healthy Samoa's Smoothie

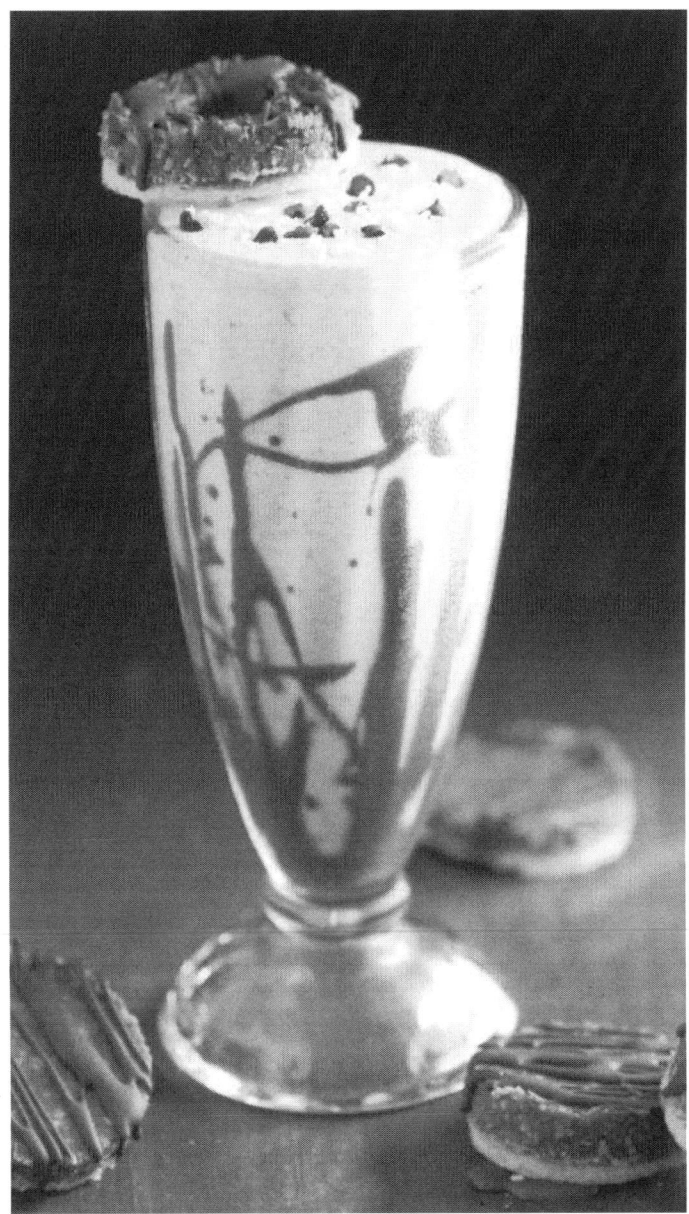

Prep time: 10mins

Total time: 10mins

Servings: 2

Ingredients:

- 1 tablespoon of homemade chocolate syrup

- 1 cup unsweetened almond milk and vanilla
- tablespoons of homemade caramel sauce with dates (or classic caramel sauce)
- ½ teaspoon of vanilla extract
- tablespoons (packed) of coconut flour
- Packages of natural sweetener (stevia, Truvia, etc.)
- 1 tablespoon of chia seeds
- 1 cup of ice cubes

Instructions:

1. Drizzle 2 glasses with chocolate syrup and place the smoothie in the freezer.
2. In a high-speed mixer (I used my Vitamix), add all ingredients except ice. Blend until smoothly.
3. Add the ice and mix until smooth. Add more ice for a thick shake texture. Serve immediately or cool later.

Nutritional values:

- Calories: 120 kcal
- Fat: 4 g
- Sodium: 105 mg
- Carbohydrates: 17 g
- Protein: 4 g
- Calcium: 250 mg
- Iron: 1.1 mg

68. Healthy raspberry thumbprint cookies

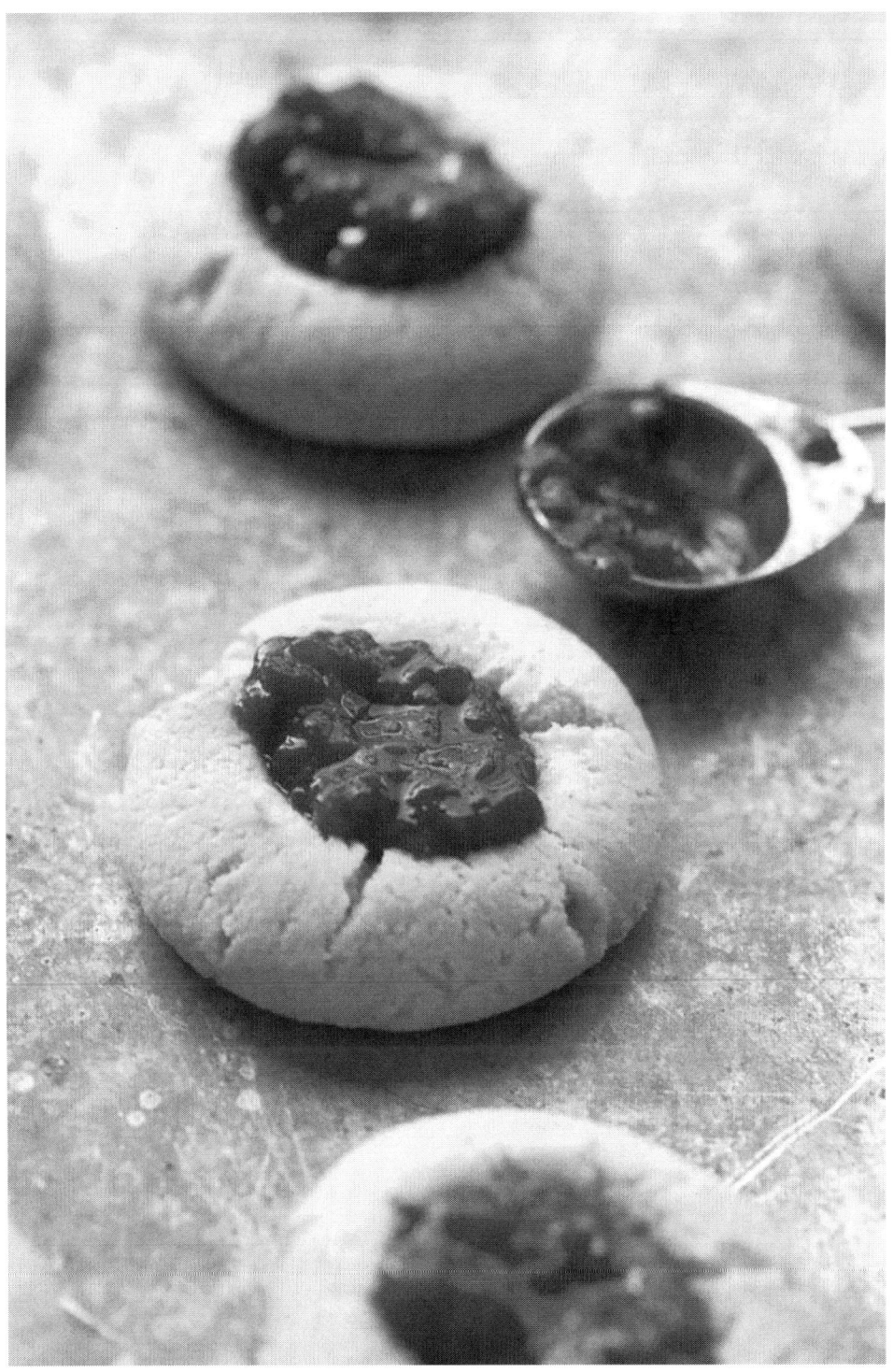

Prep time: 20mins

Cook time: 10mins

Total time: 30mins

Servings: 12 cookies

Ingredients:

- Cups + 2 tablespoons (300 g) all-purpose flour
- 1/4 teaspoon salt
- 1 cup (226g) unsalted butter, chilled and diced into 1-tablespoon pieces
- 2/3 cup (140g) granulated sugar
- 1/2 teaspoon of almond extract
- 1/2 cup seedless raspberry jam

Glaze (optional)

- 1 cup (124g) caster sugar
- 1 teaspoon of almond extract
- 4 teaspoons of water

Preparations:

1. Preheat the oven to 350 ° F (180 ° C). In a bowl mix the flour and salt, set aside.
2. In the big bowl of an electric stand mixer fitted with the paddle attachment, whisk together the butter and sugar until just combined (it will take a minute or two since the butter is cold).
3. Mix in the almond extract and then add the flour mixture until the mixture is just mixed (it will take a bit of mixing as the butter is cold so be patient, it will seem dry and crumbly at first).
4. Roll into 1-inch balls, about 1 tablespoon each, and place 2 inches apart on ungreased baking sheets.
5. Make a small notch with your thumb or forefinger on each cookie (large enough to fit 1/4 - 1/2 teaspoon of jam). Fill each one with 1/4 - 1/2 teaspoon of jam.
6. Chill in the refrigerator for at least 20 minutes (or in the freezer for 10 minutes). Bake in preheated oven for 14-18 minutes.
7. Cool several minutes on a baking sheet, and then transfer to a wire rack to cool.
8. For the frosting: Whisk together all the frosting ingredients in a small bowl, adding enough water to reach the desired consistency.
9. Pour or toss the mixture into a sandwich-sized resealable bag, cut a small tip off one corner, and drizzle over chilled cookies. Let stand at room temperature and then store in an airtight container.

Nutritional values:

- Calories: 259.3 kcal (13.5%)
- Carbohydrates: 19.59 g (6.3%)
- Proteins: 4.15 g (8.7%)

- Fibers: 5.77 g (19.2%)
- Fats: 16.98 g (31.9%)

69. Healthy blueberry lemon ricotta parfaits

Prep time: 20mins

Total time: 20mins

Servings: 4

Ingredients:

- 16 ounces skim ricotta cheese
- tablespoons lemon juice
- 1 tablespoon lemon zest
- 1 teaspoon of liquid stevia extract
- cups fresh blueberry

Instructions:

1. Add the ricotta, lemon juice, lemon zest, and stevia extract to the blender. Puree until it is completely smooth and airy.
2. Add some blueberries to the bottom of 4 perfect glass cups, then layer on the ricotta fluff. Keep the two going until everything is used up. Cover and chill for 3 or more hours.
3. Serve with whipped cream and extra blueberries, or as it is. Enjoy!

Nutritional values:

- Calories: 190 kcal
- Fat: 10 g
- Cholesterol: 50 mg
- Sodium: 160 mg
- Carbohydrates: 15 g
- Protein: 13 g
- Vitamin C: 12.4 mg
- Calcium: 300 mg

70. Healthy chocolate chip cookies

Preparation time: 20mins

Total time: 20mins

Servings: 14 cookies

Ingredients:

Dry ingredients:

- ¾ cup spelled flour (100 g)
- ½ cup almond flour (45 g)
- ½ tsp chemical yeast (baking powder)
- ¼ tsp salt

Wet Ingredients:

- tbsp coconut oil (25 g, melted)
- ¼ cup honey (60 g)
- 1 large egg, at room temperature
- 1 tsp vanilla extract

Others:

- 1 cup chocolate chips (100 g)

Instructions:

Dry ingredients:

- Add all the dry ingredients to a bowl and mix well. Reserve.

Wet Ingredients:

1. Add the coconut oil and honey to another bowl and beat for 1-2 minutes. Then add the egg and vanilla extract. Beat well.
2. Add the dry ingredients and beat until integrated. Finally, add the chocolate chips and join everything with a spatula. The dough will be a little moist. Let it rest for at least 10 minutes so that the almond flour absorbs the moisture.
3. After 10 minutes, form the dough into balls using a 1 ½ tbsp ice cream scoop, do not compact it too much. Place on a baking sheet lined with greaseproof paper. Leave about 5 cm between them.
4. With lightly oiled fingers, press the dough to a thickness of 4 mm, more or less. Don't make them too thick as they will rise somewhat in the oven.

Baked:

1. Bake in a preheated oven at 190ºC, without a fan, in the middle part, with upper and lower heat. Bake for 10 minutes if you want the cookies to be tender. Bake a few more minutes if you prefer them crisp.
2. Remove from the oven and allow to cool completely. To enjoy!

71. Healthy key lime pie dip

Prep time: 10mins

Total time: 10mins

Servings: 4

Ingredients:

- 16 ounces cream cheese, softened
- 1/2 cup granulated sugar
- 1/4 cup milk
- 1/2 teaspoon vanilla extract
- Juice and zest of two limes
- Green Colour, Optional
- Graham Crackers, for serving

Instructions:

1. In a bowl, combine cream cheese, sugar, milk, and vanilla with a hand mixer, until well combined.
2. Mix the juice and zest of both limes and green food coloring if using. Serve immediately with graham crackers, or chill until ready to use.

Nutritional values:

- Calories: 100 kcal
- Fat: 3 g
- Cholesterol: 15 mg
- Sodium: 450 mg
- Carbohydrates: 6 g
- Proteins: 13 g
- Calcium: 40 mg
- Iron: 1.8 mg

72. Healthy oatmeal raisin cookies

Ingredients:

- 1 cup oatmeal (40 g)
- 1 cup of wheat flour (120 g)
- ¼ cup of stevia or honey (60 g)
- ½ cup of oil (125 mL)

- 1 tablespoon of baking powder (15 g)
- Some eggs
- 1 cup of raisins (150 g)

Preparation:

1. Put all the dry ingredients into a bowl. That is oats, wheat flour, stevia (or honey), and a tablespoon of baking powder.
2. Add the eggs and with a whisk, begin to mix vigorously.
3. Slow down the beat and little by little, pour the oil into the mixture. Keep whisking the ingredients.
4. Look at the consistency of the dough that remains. If you notice it a bit lacking in thickness, add a little of each of the ingredients. If you see that it is too thick, rigid, pour water little by little and beat until you achieve the consistency you need.
5. Make sure to sweeten it with stevia or honey. In case you want to be sweeter, you can vary the amounts of these ingredients. Ready the dough, pour the contents into the cookie mold, and complete the tray that will go to the oven until you finish.
6. Almost to finish, place the raisins on each of the cookies on the tray.
7. Turn the oven to 180 ºC and let them cook for 25 minutes.
8. Look through the oven slit when they are lifted (for the baking powder). To know when they are ready, stick the tip of a knife. If it comes out dry, they are ready to eat.
9. Finally, remove from the oven, let them cool for a few minutes and enjoy them in the company of a hot coffee, chocolate, or a glass of warm milk. Delicious!

Nutritional values:

- Calories: 207 kcal
- Fat: 8 g
- Cholesterol: 28 mg
- Sodium: 86 mg
- Potassium: 180 mg
- Carbohydrates: 30 g
- Protein: 3 g
- Calcium: 40 mg
- Iron: 1.2 mg

73. Healthy Black Velvet Chia Seed Pudding

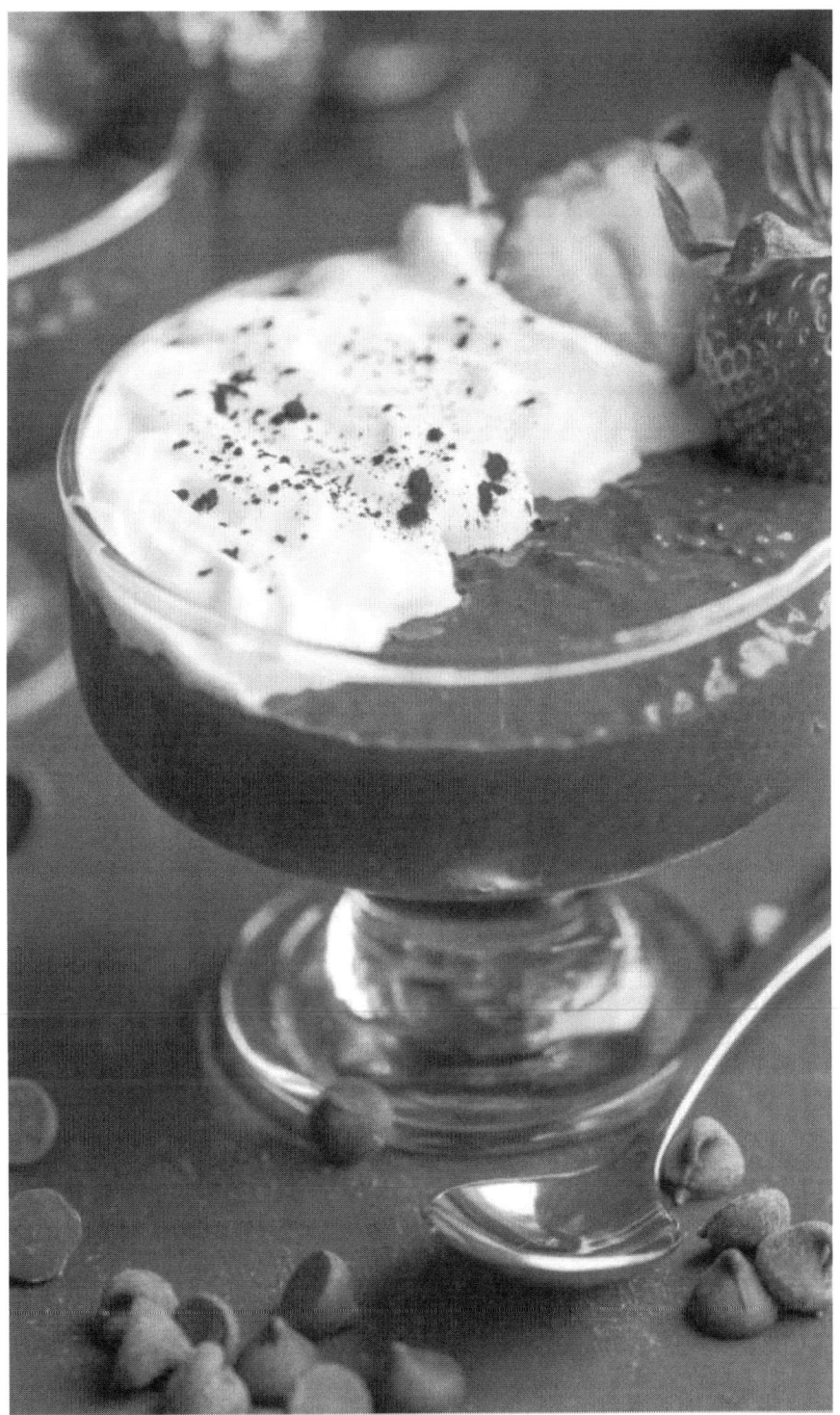

Prep time: 5mins

Total time: 5mins

Servings: 3

Ingredients:

- 36 g (3 tablespoons) of chia seeds
- 10 g (2 tablespoons) processed unsweetened Dutch cocoa powder
- Packages of natural sweetener
- Pinch of salt
- ¾ cup + 2 tablespoons unsweetened almond milk and vanilla
- Tablespoons of roasted beet puree (see this post for instructions)
- 1 teaspoon vanilla extract

Instructions:

1. Add the chia seeds, cocoa powder, sweetener, and salt to the shaker. Pour in a 1/2 cup of milk. Cover and shake vigorously with the cap.
2. Add the rest of the milk, the beet purée, and the vanilla extract and shake again. Pour in the jars evenly, seal tightly and refrigerate overnight.
3. Serve and have fun the next morning!

Nutritional values:

- Calories: 130 kcal
- Fat: 9 g
- Sodium: 140 mg
- Carbohydrates: 13 g
- Protein: 6 g
- Calcium: 350 mg
- Iron: 3.6 mg

74. Healthy Cake Batter Milkshake

Prep time: 10mins

Total time: 10mins

Servings: 3

Ingredients:

- 2 cups of low-fat plain kefir
- 2 cups crushed ice
- ½ cup of old-fashioned rolled oats
- 1 teaspoon of vanilla paste
- 1 teaspoon of natural butter flavor

- Stevia liquid extract ½ tsp (to taste)
- ½ teaspoon of Almond Extract
- Natural rainbow not equal

Instructions:

1. Put all the ingredients in the blender and purée until smooth. Give the taste and add the sweetener/ice / etc. To taste it.
2. Pour in the serving glasses. Serve with natural whipped cream (avoid brands that use hydrogenated oils,) and natural confetti or straws alone!

Nutritional values:

- Calories: 140 kcal
- Fat: 3 g
- Cholesterol: 15 mg
- Sodium: 100 mg
- Carbohydrates: 21 g
- Protein: 8 g
- Calcium: 200 mg
- Iron: 1.1 mg

75. Healthy Pumpkin Ice Cream

Ingredients:

- 1 kg of diced pumpkin
- Cups (tea) sugar
- Cloves (or cloves)
- Cinnamon sticks
- 1 can of sour cream

Preparation:

1. Cook the pumpkin with sugar, cloves, and cinnamon over low heat (160 ºC).
2. If necessary, add a little water.
3. Remove from heat, discard cloves and cinnamon, and mash until pureed.
4. Beat the cream until fluffy.
5. Add the pumpkin and beat well.
6. Freeze for 6 hours.

Nutritional values:

- Calories: 204 kcal
- Fat: 15 g
- Sugar: 15 g
- Carbohydrates: 16 g
- Fibers: 0.6 g
- Protein: 2 g
- Cholesterol: 47 mg

76. Baked oatmeal à la Pumpkin Pie

Ingredients:

- 100 g of pumpkin puree (purchased or homemade, for example, from Hokkaido)
- 50 g of butter
- 1 egg (ML)
- 75 g of raw cane sugar (for example, dark muscovado)
- 1 teaspoon cinnamon
- 1/2 teaspoon ground ginger
- 1/4 teaspoon ground nutmeg
- 1/4 teaspoon ground cloves
- 1 pinch of fine sea salt
- 200 ml of milk
- 150 g of thick oats

Preparation:

1. Since the oatmeal has to steep for several hours, it is best to prepare the mixture the evening before and only put it in the oven for baking in the morning. If you can't get unseasoned pumpkin puree, you can easily make it yourself. To do this, cut a small Hokkaido pumpkin with the skin into thin slices (remove the seeds etc. beforehand) and bake in the oven at 180 ° C for 20-30 minutes. Puree with a hand blender or the food processor while still warm.
2. Melt the butter in a small saucepan and set aside for a few minutes to cool. Put the egg, brown sugar, and spices in a bowl and stir well. Add the pumpkin puree and milk and stir until smooth. If the pumpkin puree is very dry, it is best to mix it with the milk first to avoid lumps. Finally, mix in the oat flakes and cover, and leave to soak in the refrigerator for several hours.
3. Preheat the oven to 180 ° C. Grease a brownie baking pan or square baking dish (about 20 x 20 cm) or line it with baking paper. Stir the oatmeal porridge well again, then pour it into the prepared dish and smooth it out with the back of a spoon. Bake on medium-high for 40-45

minutes until the flakes are crispy and golden brown. Take out of the oven, cut into square pieces and enjoy while warm with cold milk.

Nutritional values:

- Calories: 270 kcal
- Protein: 4 g
- Fat: 18 g
- Carbohydrates: 21 g

77. Pumpkin spiced macarons

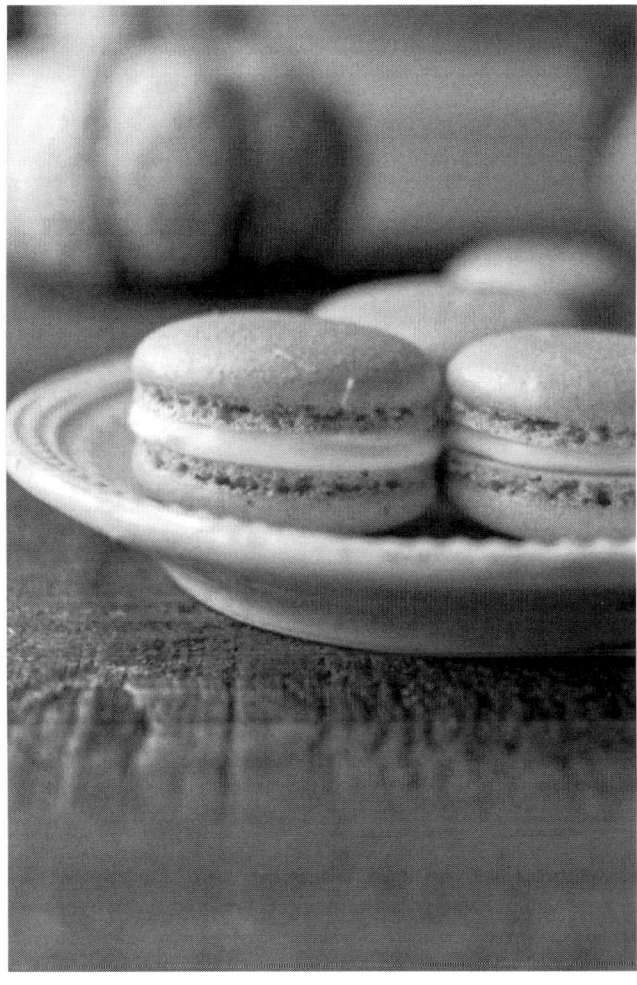

Ingredients:

For the meringue:

- 100 g of ground almonds
- 100 g of powdered sugar
- 35 ml of water

- 100 g of granulated sugar
- 35 g + 35 g of egg whites at room temperature
- 1 teaspoon of orange dye powder
- 1 teaspoon of cinnamon
- 1 teaspoon of nutmeg

For the filling:

- 150 gr of pumpkin pulp
- g of agar-agar
- 1 egg
- 50 g of sugar
- gr of corn-starch
- 70 g of butter
- 1 teaspoon of cinnamon
- 1 teaspoon of nutmeg

Instructions:

1. Pour the ground almonds and icing sugar into the food processor. Operate for about 30 seconds. Then pass the mixture through a sieve.
2. Put the sugar and water in a saucepan. Mix with a spatula to mix the ingredients well. Heat the mixture on the stove until it reaches 118 ° C. While the sugar is cooking, put the first egg white (35 g) in the mixer. When the mixture of water and sugar has reached 114 ° C, turn on the planetary mixer (used a high speed) and start whipping the egg white.
3. When the syrup reaches 118 ° C, reduce the speed and add it to the egg white little by little. Continue to beat the egg whites and add the orange coloring. Whip until you get a smooth and shiny meringue.
4. Put the second egg white in a bowl and add the mix of almond flour and icing sugar. Mix with a spatula to incorporate all the ingredients well. You will need to get a very thick mixture.
5. Gradually add the whipped egg white. You will need to obtain a homogeneous, semi-liquid mixture. Transfer the mixture to a piping bag. Line the pan with parchment paper and create small balls of meringue. When you have filled all the plate, beat it vigorously on the work surface to smooth the surface of the macarons. Using a sieve, spread the nutmeg mixed with cinnamon over the surface of the macarons.
6. Cook the shells in the preheated oven at 160 ° C for about 12 minutes. When cooked, remove them from the oven and let them cool.
7. Prepare the cream: cook the pumpkin in the oven for about 25/30 minutes. Reduce it to pulp and pass it through a sieve.

8. Put the egg and sugar mixed with the corn-starch in a saucepan. Beat lightly with a whisk. Add the pumpkin pulp, cinnamon, and nutmeg. Stir and put the saucepan on low heat. Add the butter cut into small pieces and as soon as it reaches a boil, add the agar-agar. Continue to cook the mixture for a couple of minutes, continuing to mix with a spatula. Transfer the cream to a bowl and let it cool completely. Then put it in the fridge for at least 2/3 hours.
9. Assemble the macarons: put the cream in a pastry bag. Fill the first half of the shells evenly and then close them with the second. Keep the macarons in the fridge for a few days.

Nutritional values:

- Calories: 90 kcal
- Carbohydrates: 12 g
- Protein: 1 g
- Fat: 4.5 g
- Sodium: 40 mg
- Potassium: 9 mg

78. Homemade Chocolate Chip Cookies Recipe

Prep time: 15mins

Total time: 15mins,

Servings: 4 cups

Ingredients:

- Cups of Flour (280 grams)
- Units of Eggs
- 1 cup of chocolate chips
- 1 cup of sugar (200 grams)
- 1 cup of Butter (225 grams)
- 1 teaspoon baking powder

Steps to follow to make this recipe:

1. Take a container and mix well the butter with the sugar to start making homemade cookies.
2. Then add the eggs and continue to beat. Once integrated, add the previously sifted flour with the baking powder and mix until the dough is homogeneous.
3. Finally, add the chocolate chips and mix with a spoon, a spatula, or your hands in the batter. You can leave the dough in the refrigerator for 20 minutes and knead it again for 3 minutes when you remove it. It will achieve greater consistency in this way.

Shape and place your cookies on the baking sheet, with some separation. Bake the chocolate chip cookies for 20 minutes.

79. Pumpkin swirl brownies

Prep time: 30mins

Cook time: 45mins

Total time: 60mins

Ingredients:

- Tablespoons (1 stick) unsalted butter, plus more for the skillet
- Ounces bittersweet chocolate, chopped
- Cups all-purpose flour
- 1 teaspoon of baking powder
- 1/4 teaspoon cayenne pepper
- 1/2 teaspoon salt
- 1 3/4 cups sugar
- Large eggs
- 1 tablespoon pure vanilla extract
- 1 1/4 cups solid pumpkin
- 1/4 cup vegetable oil
- 1 teaspoon ground cinnamon
- 1/4 teaspoon ground nutmeg
- 1/2 cup chopped hazelnuts or other nuts

Instructions:

1. Preheat the oven to 350 degrees. Butter a 9-inch square baking pan or plate. Line bottom of skillet with parchment paper; butter lining.
2. Melt the chocolate and butter in a heat-proof bowl set over a saucepan of water over low heat, stirring occasionally until smooth.
3. In a large bowl, combine flour, baking powder, cayenne pepper, and salt; set aside. Place the sugar, eggs, and vanilla in a bowl of an electric blender with the paddle attachment; beat until fluffy and well blended, 3 to 5 minutes. Whisk in a mixture of flour.
4. Divide the batter into 2 medium bowls (about 2 cups per bowl). Stir the chocolate mixture in a bowl. In another bowl, add the pumpkin, oil, cinnamon, and nutmeg. Transfer half of the chocolate mass to the top of the prepared saucepan with a rubber spatula. Top with half of the

pumpkin batter. Repeat to make 1 more layer of chocolate and 1 more layer of pumpkin. Work fast so batters don't notice.

5. Using a small spatula or table knife, gently swirl the 2 batters to create a marble effect. Sprinkle with walnuts.
6. Bake until done, 40 to 45 minutes. Let cool in a skillet on a wire rack. Cut into 16 squares.

80. Chocolate peanut squares

Preparation time: 10 minutes

Total time: 2 hours, 10 minutes

Ingredients:

- 100 g dark chocolate with a minimum of 70% cocoa solids
- 4 tbsp butter or coconut oil
- 1 pinch salt
- 60 ml peanut butter
- ½ tsp vanilla extract
- 1 tsp powdered licorice or ground cardamom (green)
- 60 ml (35 g) chopped salted peanuts, for decoration

Instructions:

1. Melt the chocolate and butter or coconut oil in the microwave or a water-bath pot. If you don't have a pot for a water bath, you can put a glass bowl on top of a pot with boiling water. Make sure the water does not reach the container. The chocolate will melt by the heat of the steam. Mix all other ingredients and pour the mixture into a small roasting pan lined with baking paper (no larger than 10 x 15 centimeters).
2. Let cool for a while and cover with finely chopped peanuts or other creative toppings. Refrigerate.
3. When the dough is ready, cut it into small squares with a sharp knife. Remember that all whims are small, not more than a square of 2.5 cm x 2.5 cm. Store in the refrigerator or freezer.

Nutritional values:

- Calories: 120 kcal
- Fat: 4 g
- Sodium: 105 mg
- Carbohydrates: 17 g
- Protein: 4 g
- Calcium: 250 mg

- Iron: 1.1 mg

81. Nougat Whims

Ingredients:

- 210 g dark chocolate with at least 70% cocoa solids
- 125 ml (110 g) coconut oil, divided
- 400 g coconut milk, only the solid part
- Tbsp peanut butter or any other nut butters you like
- 1 tbsp (5 g) cocoa powder
- 1 teaspoon vanilla extract

Instructions:

1. Melt half of the chocolate in a water bath or microwave over low heat. Add a quarter of coconut oil and mix well.
2. Pour into a greased mold and coated with baking paper, (approximately 13 x 20 inches, if you make 40) and let cool in the refrigerator or freezer.
3. Carefully heat the solid part of the coconut milk (canned) in a different pan. Let it simmer for a few minutes.
4. Add half of the coconut oil, nut butter, cocoa powder, and vanilla while stirring. Make a smooth mixture. If the dough separates, use a hand blender and press several times to make it uniform.
5. Remove from heat and pour over chocolate. Return the pan to the refrigerator or freezer to cool again while the rest of the chocolate melts as in step 1.
6. Add the remaining coconut oil to the chocolate and mix. Spread it in a layer over the cold nougat. Replace in the refrigerator and let stand for at least an hour, preferably longer.
7. Cut into 30-40 small pieces. Store in an airtight container in the refrigerator or freezer. The nougat is best served slightly cold.

82. Cheesecake mousse with raspberries

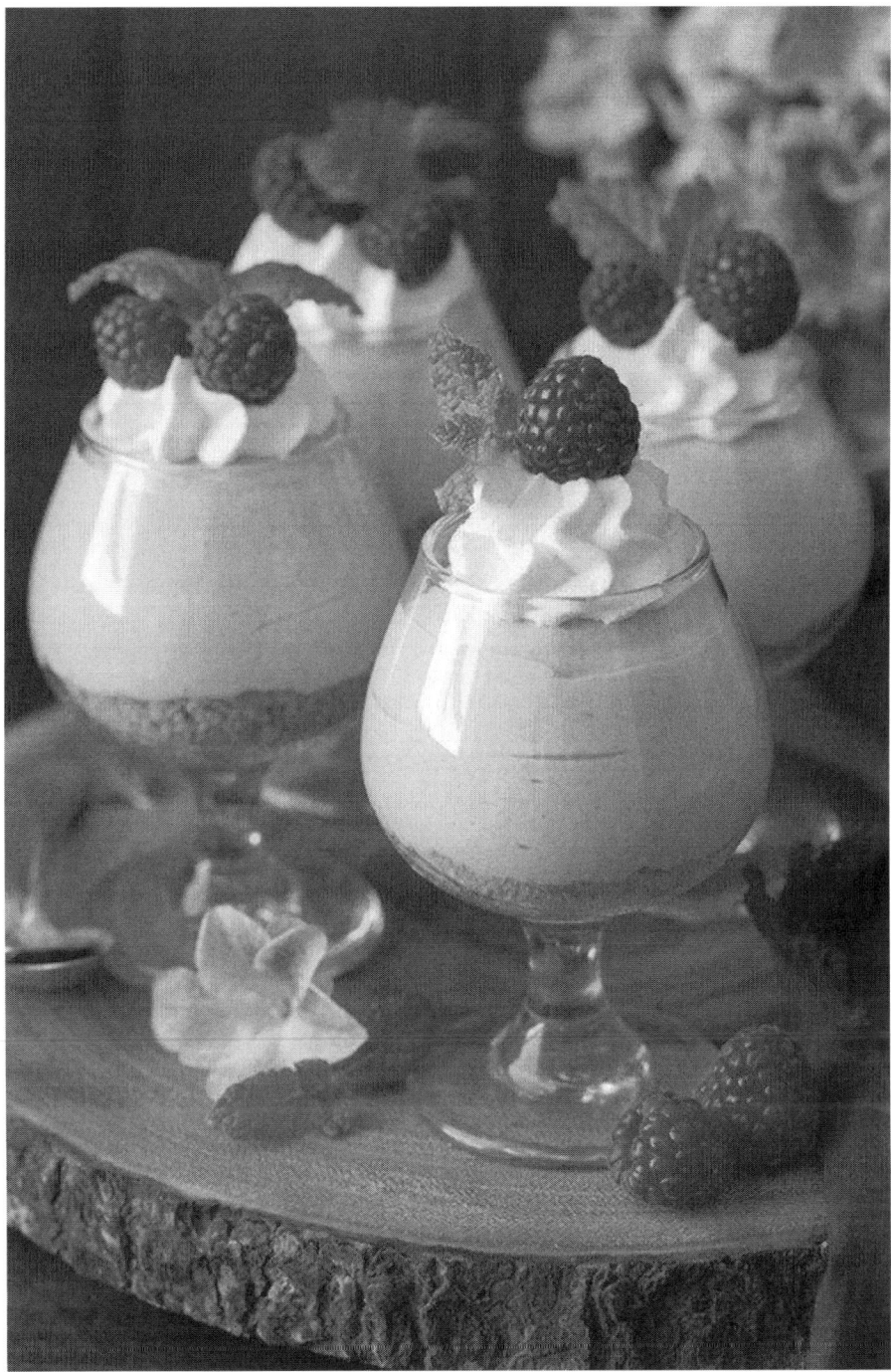

Ingredients:

- 1 cup light lemonade filling
- 1 can 8 oz cream cheese at room temperature
- 3/4 cup SPLENDA no-calorie sweetener pellets
- 1 tbsp. at t. of lemon zest

- 1 tbsp. at t. vanilla extract
- 1 cup fresh or frozen raspberries

Preparation:

1. Beat the cream cheese until it is sparkling; add 1/2 cup SPLENDA® Granules and mix until melted. Stir in lemon zest and vanilla.
2. Reserve some raspberries for decoration. Crush the rest of the raspberries with a fork and mix them with 1/4 cup SPLENDA pellets until they are melted.
3. Lightly add the lump and cheese filling, and then gently but quickly add crushed raspberries. Share this mousse in 6 ramekins with a spoon and keep in the refrigerator until tasting.
4. Garnish mousses with reserved raspberries and garnish with fresh mint before serving.

CHAPTER 9: SALAD RECIPES

83. Chickpea salad

This recipe for legume salad is rich in iron, calcium, potassium, protein, and vitamins. It is a recipe super nutritious and very easy to prepare which can bring us a lot of energy. Also, chickpeas have a lot of serotonin, so they can help us improve our mood. Departure information:

- *2 people*
- *Level of difficulty: Very easy*
- *Time preparation: 15 minutes*

Ingredients:

- 1 unit (s) of garlic (one tooth)
- 1 unit (s) of chickpeas
- 1 unit (s) of onion medium
- 1 unit (s) of red pepper
- 1 pinch of paprika
- 1 pinch of pepper
- 1 pinch of parsley (one bunch)
- 1 pinch of salt (optional)
- 1 glass of vinegar
- 1 glass of olive oil
- 1 unit (s) of green pepper
- 400 grams of canned Garbanzo
- 1 tablespoon lemon juice

Preparation:

1. Chop all the red peppers, Green pepper, onion, and parsley and mix them with the chickpeas.
2. In a separate glass mix an abundant stream of oil, another stream of vinegar, lemon juice, a teaspoon of paprika (sweet), a pinch of pepper, a clove of garlic, chopped into small pieces, and a little salt (optional).
3. Add the canned Garbanzo
4. Then add the dressing to the vegetables.

Nutritional facts for 100 grs:

Composition	Amount (gr)	CDR (%)

Calories:	511.42	26.7%
Carbohydrates:	37.33	12%
Proteins:	16.66	34.8%
Fibers:	11.54	38.5%
Fat:	31.84	59.9%

84. Salad with Avocado, Pineapple and Cucumbers

Time preparation: 25 min.

Servings: 4

Ingredients:

- 1 sliced cucumber
- Slices of pineapple
- 1/2 red onion filleted
- Avocados
- 1/3 cup olive oil
- Tbsp. lemon juice
- 1 cdita salt
- 1 cdita pepper

Preparation:

1. Cut the avocado and pineapple into medium cubes.
2. Subsequently cut the cucumber along, remove the seeds with a spoon and cut into slices.
3. Mix the above in a bowl, add the red onion, salt, pepper, and season with olive oil and lemon juice.

Nutritional facts:

- Calories: 90.2 kcal
- Total Fat: 4.6 g
- Dietary Fiber: 2.5 g
- Saturated Fat: 1.7 g

85. Mango with avocado salad

Time preparation: 10 minutes

Servings: 4 people

Ingredients:

- 1 unit (s) of chopped lettuce
- 1 pinch of pepper
- 1 unit (s) of avocado
- 1 unit (s) of mango
- 1 tablespoon white wine vinegar
- 1 tablespoon of olive oil
- 2 tablespoon of chopped toasted almonds
- 2 tablespoon dried cranberries
- Salt

Preparation:

1. Peel and chop the vegetables.
2. Put the lettuce, mango, avocado, almonds, and cranberries in a bowl.
3. On the other hand, mix the oil with the vinegar and add salt and pepper.
4. Pour over the salad and mix.
5. Serve on plates and enjoy.

Nutritional facts for 100 grs:

Composition	Amount (gr)	CDR (%)
Calories:	259.3	13.5%
Carbohydrates:	19.59	6.3%
Proteins:	4.15	8.7%
Fibers:	5.77	19.2%
Fat:	16.98	31.9%

86. Avocado and lettuce salad

The avocado is good for lowering cholesterol and contains healthy fats, fiber, and many vitamins, while lettuce has almost no calories and has many properties. Departure information:

- *Time preparation: 10 minutes*
- *Servings: 2 people*

Ingredients:

- 1 unit (s) of tomato cut
- 1 unit (s) of lettuce
- 0.5 unit (s) of red pepper, diced julienne
- 1 pinch of pepper
- 1 unit (s) of avocado
- 2 tablespoon nuez chopped (walnut crepes)
- 1 pinch of salt
- 2 tablespoon of Modena balsamic vinegar
- 2 tablespoon of lemon juice
- 1 pinch of extra virgin olive oil

Preparation:

1. Wash the lettuce well and chop it.
2. Wash and chop the remaining ingredients such as the Tomato, red pepper or diced julienne, Avocado, Nuez chopped, Modena balsamic vinegar.
3. Mix the lemon juice, vinegar, virgin oil, salt, and pepper. Then toss on the salad.
4. Remove and add the nuts (optional) to garnish.

Nutritional composition for 100 grs:

Composition	Amount (gr)	CDR (%)
Calories:	315.53	16.5%
Carbohydrates:	10.8	3.5%
Proteins:	6.55	13.7%
Fibers:	7.55	25.2%
Fat:	25.88	48.7%

87. Vegan Vegetable Mini Tortillas

Time preparation: 50 minutes

Servings: 4 people

Ingredients:

- 1 unit (s) of zucchini
- 1 unit (s) of onion
- 2 unit (s) of carrot
- 1 pinch of pepper
- 1 teaspoon parsley
- 1 pinch of salt
- 2 unit (s) of potato small
- 1 tablespoon of olive oil
- 1 pinch of Comino
- 2 tablespoon of chickpea flour

Preparation:

This recipe for Vegan Vegetable Mini Tortillas is a very tasty and healthy recipe that will surprise you. Also, the fact of being made only with vegetable ingredients makes it suitable for vegans but also very healthy to be low in vegetable fats (as long as we take care to cook them with little oil). There goes the recipe:

1. Peel potatoes, onions, and carrots. Wash the zucchini and cut all the vegetables into as small as possible (in brunoise).
2. In a pan fry all the vegetables with a little oil until they are very soft. Add salt, Comino, pepper, and a few sprigs of chopped parsley and leave over medium heat.
3. We undo the chickpea flour in a little water. It has to be a texture like a beaten egg, so we will be adding the water little by little until it is almost liquid. We add it to the pan of the vegetables without stopping to stir until it is fully integrated. There will be a paste that can be worked with your hands.
4. When the mixture has cooled a little, and we can work by hand, we flour our hands and make balls twice the size of a meatball. Then we flatten them a bit to give them a hamburger shape, and we put them on the griddle with a drop of oil on both sides.
5. And ready! The vegan vegetable omelets are ready to serve.

Nutritional composition for 100 grs:

Composition	Amount (gr)	CDR (%)
Calories:	196.09	10.2%
Carbohydrates:	25.4	8.2%
Proteins:	6.92	14.5%

88. Broccoli Soup, Green Leaves, And Beans

Green soup of vegetables and beans, perfect for a quick dinner or a light lunch.

Time preparation: 50 min

Servings: 6 people

Ingredients:

- 1 tablespoon of olive oil
- 1/2 medium-size onion, cut into large pieces
- 3 cloves of garlic in pieces
- 1 teaspoon of salt
- 1 medium-size broccoli head in pieces
- 6 cups of water
- 1 spinach bunches or 3 large fleas of green leaves kale, spinach, etc.
- 1 fist of coriander leaves and stems
- 11/2 cups white beans cooked beans
- Freshly ground black pepper
- 2-3 tablespoons fresh chopped dill
- Lemon juice to serve

Preparation:

1. Place a large pot and a lid over medium heat and add the tablespoon of olive oil, onion, garlic, and half a teaspoon salt. Leave for 5-7 minutes or until the onion is transparent.
2. Add the broccoli and leave for about five minutes until they change color and start to brown slightly.
3. Add water and spinach. Cover and let it begin to boil over low heat.

4. When the broccoli is soft add the cilantro fist, the dill (if you are going to use it), and the beans.
5. Blend very carefully with a food processor or in the blender. Check salt and add black pepper.
6. Before serving, squeeze the juice of a lemon. You can put lemons on the table so that everyone can put more to their liking.

Nutritional Facts:

- Calories: 34 kcal
- Carbohydrate: 6.6 g
- Fibers: 2.6 g
- Sugar: 1.7 g
- Fat: 0.4 g
- Protein: 2.8 g

89. Baked omelet with baby spinach

Spinach is a vegetable plant belonging to the family Chenopodiaceous, native to Southwest Asia. It is a vegetable that consumes the triangular leaves cooked a beautiful green color. They must be washed carefully because they usually contain a lot of soil in their folds. Spinach brings a lot of pro-vitamin A and an interesting amount of iodine. Contrary to popular belief, spinach contains little iron, and the body poorly assimilates it.

Time preparation: 30mins

Ingredients:

- 200 grams of spinach
- Two units of Egg
- Two slices of mozzarella cheese
- Parmesan cheese
- 3tsp of Butter
- One pinch of Salt and Pepper

Preparations:

1. Before making this delicious tortilla, the first step is to prepare all the ingredients.
2. In a pot with boiling water, add the previously washed spinach and cook approximately 4 minutes.
3. Once the spinach is ready, dry them one by one as much as possible and cut them a little. Then, mix with the beaten eggs and season with salt and pepper.
4. To butter with a refractory one to avoid that the tortilla sticks. Add half of the spinach and cover with mozzarella cheese, Parmesan cheese slices.

5. To finish the tortilla, add the rest of the spinach and cover with the grated Parmesan cheese. Bake it at 180º C. And time for about 15 minutes until browned.
6. Once the spinach omelet is ready, wait for it to cool a bit and unmold. It can be consumed cold or hot, ideal as a side dish of a beef loin.

Nutritional information:

- Calories: 240.8 kcal
- Total Fat: 17.6 g
- Total Carbohydrate: 5.1 g
- Dietary Fiber: 1.3 g
- Sugars: 0.5 g
- Protein: 15.5 g

90. Vegetarian recipe

The perfect salad for families, parties, potlucks, and BBQs. Make it advancing of time and relax before it's time to eat.

Time preparation: 1 hour

Ingredients:

- 1 cup of green beans
- 2 carrots
- Sweet corn
- Cooked rice
- A teaspoon of mustard
- A little honey
- Olive oil
- A handful of cooked chickpeas
- Three or four chopped pistachios

Preparation:

1. You have to mix some green beans and some boiled or steamed carrots, along with sweet corn and cooked rice.
2. To dress it, mix a teaspoon of mustard with a little honey and olive oil. And if you want to turn it into a complete and balanced single dish, you can add a handful of cooked chickpeas and three or four chopped pistachios. Besides being delicious, this vegetarian recipe is one of the best meals to take to work.

Nutritional information:

- Calories: 111 kcal
- Total Fat: 2 g
- Saturated Fat: 1 g
- Cholesterol: 10 mg
- Sodium: 58 mg
- Carbohydrates: 19 g
- Fiber: 0 g
- Sugar: 18 g
- Calcium: 15%
- Iron: 0%

91. Raw Vegetables. Chopped Salad

A fresh, crispy, and spicy way to eat the rainbow. The perfect salad for families, parties, potlucks, and BBQs. Make it advancing of time and relax before it's time to eat.

Preparation time: 15 minutes

Total time: 15 minutes

Ingredients:

- Chopped raw veggie salad
- 1 orange pepper (minced) (about 1 cup)
- 1 yellow pepper (small cut) (about 1 cup)
- 5-8 radishes (halve and cut into thin slices) (about 3/4 cup)
- small head of broccoli (minced) (about 2 cups)
- 1 seedless cucumber (small cut) (about 2 cups)
- 1 cup of halved red seedless grapes
- 2-3 tablespoons chopped fresh dill
- 1/4 cup chopped fresh parsley
- 1/4 cup of raw peeled sunflower seeds
- 1/8 cup raw hemp hearts (peeled hemp seeds)
- Oil-free dressing
- garlic clove (chopped)
- tablespoons of red wine vinegar
- 1 tablespoon of apple cider vinegar
- Juice of 1 lemon
- 1 tbsp Dijonsenf

- 1 tbsp pure maple syrup
- 1/2 teaspoon salt (or to taste)
- 1/8 tsp pepper (or to taste)

Preparation:

1. Whisk the ingredients - Chopped raw veggie salad, 1 orange pepper, yellow pepper, radishes, small head of broccoli, seedless cucumber, halved red seedless grapes, chopped fresh dill, chopped fresh parsley, raw peeled sunflower seeds, raw hemp hearts, garlic clove, red wine vinegar, apple cider vinegar, lemon, Dijonsenf, pure maple syrup, salt, pepper. For dressing in a small bowl and set aside.
2. Combine all the salad ingredients in a large bowl.
3. Pour the dressing over the chopped vegetables and wrap well.

Nutritional information:

- Calories: 111 kcal
- Total Fat: 2 g
- Saturated Fat: 1 g
- Cholesterol: 10 mg
- Sodium: 58 mg
- Carbohydrates: 19 g
- Sugar: 18 g
- Calcium: 15%

92. Mediterranean Veggie Pita Sandwich

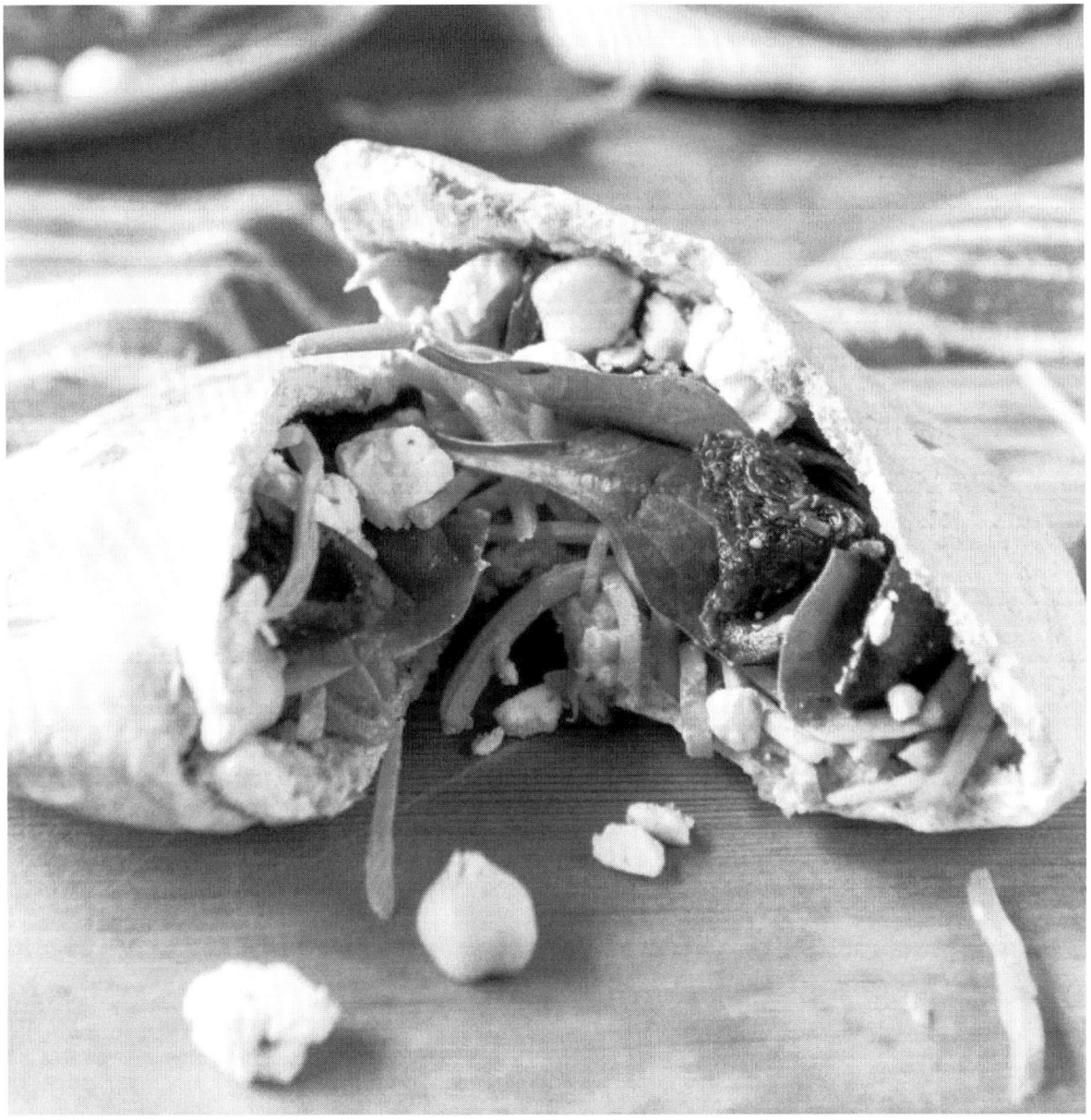

Makes 2 pita bread, can be multiplied for more portions

Time preparation: 4hours, 30mins

Ingredients:

- 1/4 cup chopped carrots
- A handful of baby spinach
- 1/4 cup chickpeas
- 1 tsp of crumbled feta cheese
- 2 tsp. of fine chopped sun-dried tomatoes

- 2 teaspoons of chopped kalamata olives
- Season with salt and pepper

Preparation:

The chopped carrots, baby spinach, chickpeas, crumbled feta cheese, chopped sun-dried tomatoes, chopped kalamata olives, salt, and pepper. Spread the bath in every pita pant. Sort the rest of the ingredients between the boxes. Eat immediately or pack in a container for lunch. Cool the device if you prepare it for more than 4 hours before eating.

Nutritional information:

- Calories: 287.6 kcal
- Sodium: 716.0 mg
- Potassium: 263.6 mg
- Total Carbohydrates: 45.7 g
- Dietary Fiber: 6.8 g

93. Classic asparagus

The asparagus classics are served with hollandaise sauce. This recipe is for the prettier ones.

Time preparation: 40 min

Ingredients for 4 servings:

- 2 kg of white asparagus
- 12 pieces of medium potatoes
- 4 eggs
- 1 first-class salt
- 1 premium sugar
- 1 tbsp butter

For the sauce:

- 200 g butter
- 2 egg yolks
- 4 tablespoons white wine
- 1 tbsp lemon juice
- 1 first-class salt
- 1 premium white pepper

Preparation:

1. Cook the peeled asparagus in plenty of hot water (seasoned with salt, sugar, and butter) for 15 - 20 minutes.
2. Peel the potatoes and cook as usual or cool with the air freezer. The eggs are cooked hard.
3. For the sauce: Dissolve the butter in a hot freezer and allow cooling slightly.
4. Grease the egg yolks with lemon juice and white wine in a warm water bath until the mass is thick.
5. Then the cooled and melted butter is slowed down slowly. Now the sauce is seasoned with salt and pepper.

Tips on the recipe: Distribute the asparagus in 4 portions and arrange with potatoes and the halved eggs on 4 plates.

Nutritional information:

- Calories: 20% daily value
- Total fat: 0.1 g (0%)
- Saturated fat: 0 g (0%)
- Total carbohydrates: 3.9 g (1%)
- Dietary fibers: 2.1 g (8%)
- Sugar: 1.9 g
- Protein: 2.2 g (4%)

94. Soup cream from palm heart

Whether winter or summer, slimming soups are always so light, healthy, and easy to digest.

They offer another benefit: they can be used during a diet to lose weight, with high levels of nutrients and calories that give the body the fullness without weight.

Time preparation: 10 mins

Ingredients:

- 250 g pupunha palm
- 3 cups chicken broth tea
- 1 cup skimmed milk
- 1 tablespoon light margarine
- A grated onion
- A garlic kernel, chopped
- Two tablespoons of wheat flour
- Small salt

Preparation:

1. Onions and garlic must be sweetened in light margarine. Then add the Pupunha palm heart and pick up a little more to absorb the spice flavor.
2. It takes 2 to 3 minutes.
3. Dissolve wheat flour in chicken broth tea. Approximately 10 mins;
4. When it is lukewarm, it is time to apply the milk by adding skimmed milk. Go back to the fire for another 5 or 6 minutes. It's time to taste the salt. Serve immediately.

Yield: 6 servings (1 medium conch)

Nutritional information:

- Calories per serving: about 62 kcal

95. Broccoli Soup, Green Leaves, And Beans

Green soup of vegetables and beans, perfect for a quick dinner or a light lunch

Time preparation: 50 min

Servings: 6 people

Ingredients:

- 1 tablespoon of olive oil
- 1/2 medium-size onion, cut into large pieces
- 3 cloves of garlic in pieces
- 1 teaspoon of salt
- 1 medium-size broccoli head in pieces
- 6 cups of water
- 1 spinach bunches or 3 large fleas of green leaves kale, spinach, etc.
- 1 fist of coriander leaves and stems
- 1 1/2 cups white beans cooked beans
- Freshly ground black pepper
- 2-3 tablespoons fresh chopped dill
- Lemon juice to serve

Preparation:

1. Place a large pot and a lid over medium heat and add the tablespoon of olive oil, onion, garlic, and half a teaspoon salt. Leave for 5-7 minutes or until the onion is transparent.
2. Add the broccoli and leave for about five minutes or until they change color and start to brown slightly.

3. Add water and spinach. Cover and let it begin to boil over low heat.
4. When the broccoli is soft add the coriander leaves and stems, the dill (if you are going to use it), and the beans.
5. Blend very carefully with a food processor or in the blender. Check salt and add black pepper.
6. Before serving, squeeze the juice of a lemon. You can put lemons on the table so that everyone can put more to their liking.

Nutritional Facts:

- Calories: 34 kcal
- Carbohydrate: 6.6 g
- Fiber: 2.6 g
- Sugar: 1.7 g
- Fat: 0.4 g
- Protein: 2.8 g

CHAPTER 10: SOUP AND STEW RECIPES

96. Nopal Soup

What you will need:

- 2 pounds of nopales, clean and diced
- 4 Roma tomatoes
- ¼ white onion
- 2 cloves of garlic
- 1 chipotle chili in adobo (optional)
- 3 cups of vegetable stock
- 1 tablespoon dried oregano
- Salt and pepper to taste

Optional coverages:

- Avocado
- Coriander
- Chives
- Lemon or Lime Juice

Process:

1. Cook the nopales for 20-25 minutes in boiling water with salt or until they lose their bright color and are tender to bit.
2. Place the tomatoes, onion, garlic, and chipotle in a blender glass. Blend until you get a creamy consistency.
3. Remove the nopales from the heat, drain them, and rinse them with enough cold water. Leave aside.
4. In a pot, sauté the tomato sauce for about 3 minutes.
5. Add cooked nopales and oregano to tomato broth. Let cook another 15 minutes.
6. add salt and pepper to taste.
7. Serve on soup plates and add toppings.

97. Vegetable broth without sodium

What you will need:

- 2 yellow onions, sliced
- 3 cloves garlic, minced

- 6 carrots, peeled and sliced
- 4 celery stalks, sliced
- 5 sprigs of dill
- 4 sprigs of parsley
- 4 scallions
- 10 cups of water

Process:

1. Add the onions over medium heat to a large pot and stir until the scent is released, about a minute. Add the garlic, carrots, celery, dill, parsley, and scallions and cook for about a minute until the herbs release their fragrance.
2. Add the water and allow it to boil. Low the heat, cover the pot, and cook for 45 minutes.
3. Turn off the heat and allow about 15 minutes to cool the broth.
4. Filter the broth through a sieve and freeze it into ice buckets, or pour it into glass jars if you use it immediately. It's going to stay a week or so.

98. Comforting noodle and chickpea soup

What you will need:

- 1 cup onion, diced
- 2 carrots, sliced
- 1 celery stalk, diced (optional)
- 2 medium diced potatoes
- 3 cloves garlic, minced
- ½ teaspoon dried thyme
- 4 cups of vegetable stock
- 2 cups of water
- ¼ cup chicken seasoning
- 6 ounces cooked spaghetti (noodles)
- 2 cups cooked chickpeas
- Salt and pepper to taste
- fresh cilantro chopped to taste

CONDIMENTO FOR "CHICKEN" (PREPARE 1 ¾ CUP):

- 1 ⅓ cup nutritional yeast
- 3 tablespoons onion powder
- 1 tablespoon garlic powder
- 1½ tablespoon dried basil

- 1 teaspoon oregano
- ½ teaspoon of turmeric
- 2 teaspoons sea salt

Process:

1. Sauté the onion in a medium saucepan over medium heat until it begins to soften, about 3 minutes.
2. Add the carrots, potatoes, and celery (if you are using it) and sauté for 2-3 minutes.
3. Add garlic, thyme, "chicken seasoning," vegetable stock, and water.
4. Cook over medium-low heat until all vegetables are tender, about 20 minutes.
5. Add the chickpeas and pasta.
6. Season with salt and pepper to taste.
7. Serve with some fresh cilantro on top.

99. Soup loaded with miso noodles

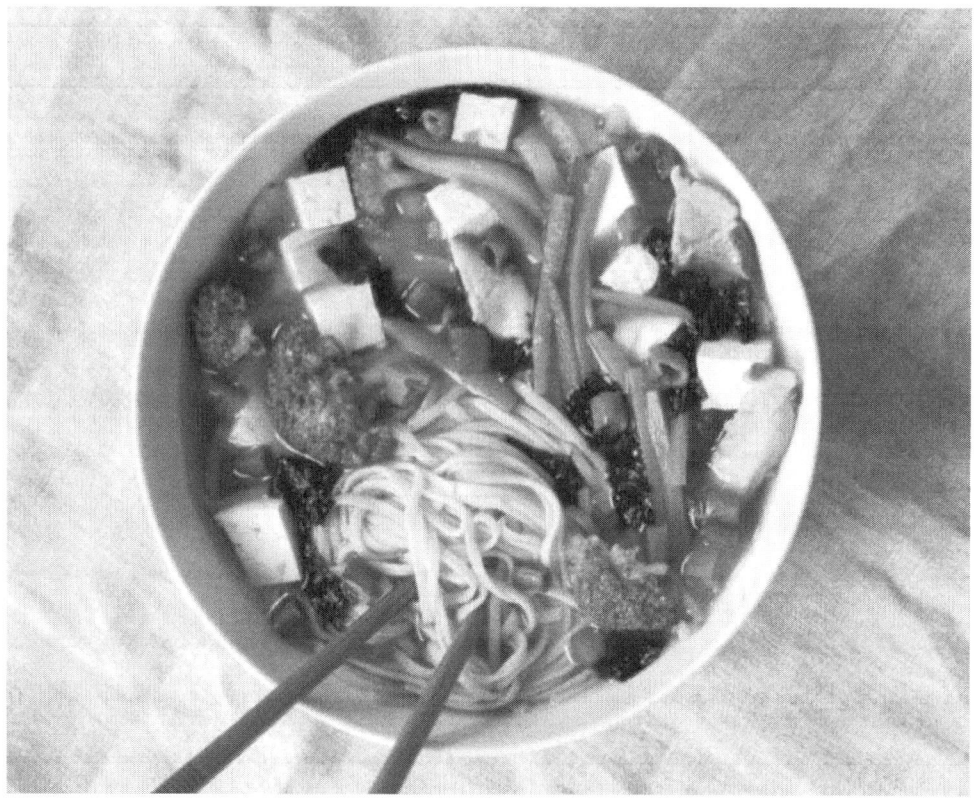

What you will need:

- 4 servings of buckwheat noodles or brown rice noodles, uncooked
- 3 cups of vegetable stock
- 3 cups of water

- 1 cup of carrot cut into julienne
- 1 cup julienne zucchini
- 1 cup thinly sliced shiitake mushrooms
- 1 cup broccoli corsages
- 3 tablespoons miso paste
- 1 package of firm tofu (14 ounces or 396 grams), cut into one-inch cubes (2.5 centimeters)
- ¼ cup chopped green onion
- 1 sheet of roasted nori seaweed, cut into pieces

Process:

1. Prepare the noodles as per the instructions for the box. Set them apart.
2. Cook the vegetable stock and water in a medium saucepan over high heat. Remove the carrots, courgettes, mushrooms, and broccoli, add heat, and cook for five minutes.
3. Use a spoon to pass to a small bowl a cup of broth. Use a fork in the broth to dissolve the miso paste and return it to the pot. Add tofu, green onions, and cooked noodles and cook for another minute until warm.
4. Move to bowls and cover with seaweed nori.

100. "Bone" mineral broth and vegetables

What you will need:

- 2 strips of 5 inches (12.7 centimeters) of dried Kombu seaweed
- 6 mushroom shiitake dry
- 6 carrots cut into pieces
- 2 medium onions cut into pieces
- 1 leek, with white and green parts, cut into pieces
- small bunch of celery, including the heart, cut into pieces
- 5 cloves of unpeeled garlic, cut in half
- 1 normal or small winter squash with peel, seeded, and cut into pieces
- 1 piece of fresh ginger 5 inches (12.7 centimeters), sliced
- 4 cups chopped vegetables, such as kale or chard
- ½ bunch fresh parsley
- 1 package of 40 g (1.4 oz) dried daikon radish (optional)

Process:

1. Combine all ingredients in a broth or large soup pot.
2. Fill the pot 2 inches (5 centimeters) below the edge with water, cover it and let it boil.

3. Remove the lid, reduce the temperature to medium/low, and let it boil for a minimum of two hours.
4. As the broth heats up, some of the water will evaporate; add more if the vegetables are exposed.
5. Cook over low heat until you can taste the delicacy of vegetables. Strain the broth and pour it into glass jars. Refrigeration works well with any broth.

101. Noodle soup with broccoli and ginger

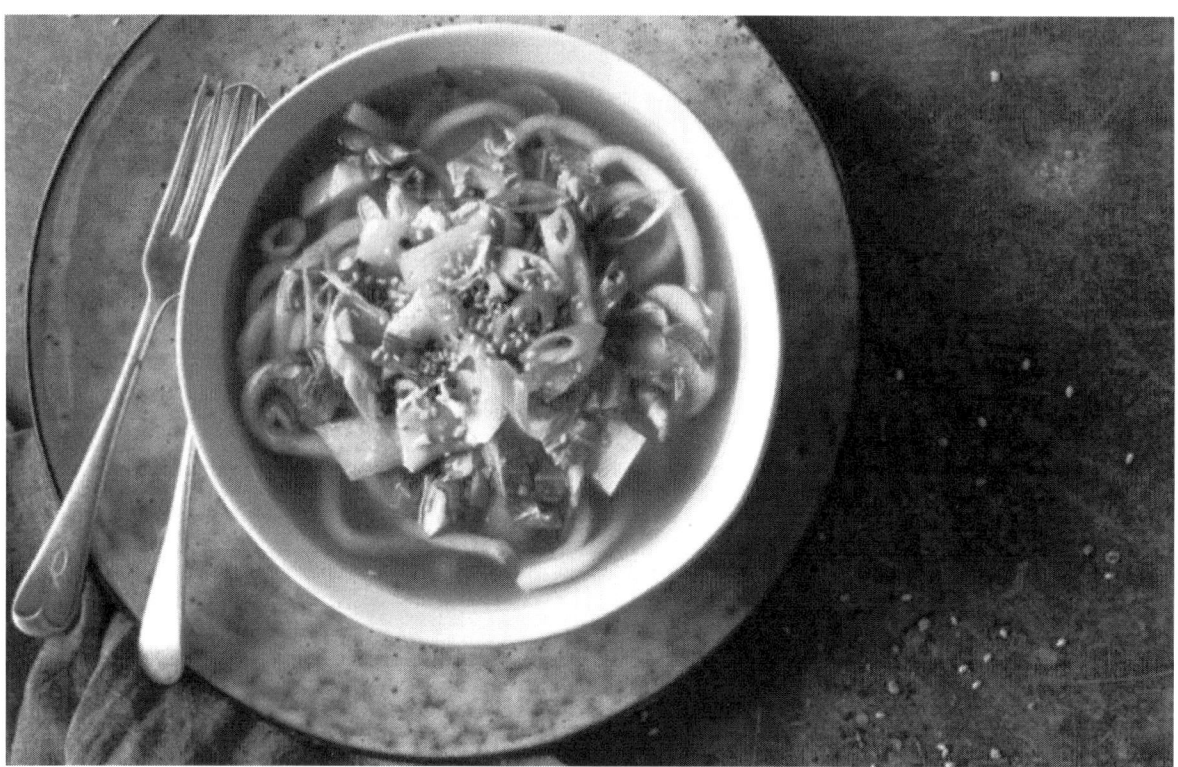

What you will need:

- 3 medium broccoli heads (7 to 8 cups)
- 1 package of small rice noodles (12 ounces or 340 g)
- 16 ounces (453 g) firm tofu, cut into ¼ to ½ inch (6 to 12 mm) cubes
- 2 pieces of two inches (5 cm) of wakame or alaria seaweed
- 4 quarts (4 liters) of water
- ¾ cup wheat-free or regular tamari
- 2 medium onions, diced (approximately 2½ cups)
- 4 tablespoons fresh ginger root, chopped or finely grated
- 3 tablespoons mirin (rice wine for cooking)
- 6 medium carrots, diced (approximately 3 cups)
- 4 medium parsnips, diced (approximately 2 cups)

Process:

1. Separate the broccoli stems from their heads. Remove the hard-outer layer of the stems and cut them into small bite-sized pieces. Set them aside. Separate broccoli headed into small pieces and set aside too.
2. Cook the noodles, strain them and let them cool. Set them aside.
3. Sauté the tofu in a non-stick skillet for 3 to 4 minutes. Add 4 teaspoons of tamari and sauté for another 3 to 4 minutes. Set it aside.
4. Place the wakame or alaria seaweed in 4 liters of water and bring it to a boil.
5. Lower the heat to medium, add the onions, and cook for 10 minutes.
6. Remove the vegetables from the sea, cut them into small pieces, and return them to the pot.
7. Add the ginger, the remaining tamari, and the peeper. Continue cooking over medium heat for 5 minutes.
8. Add carrots, parsnips, and broccoli stems. Cook for 2 minutes. Gently stir the noodles and sauteed tofu. Cook for 1 minute.
9. Add the broccoli heads. Cook over low heat until the broccoli is tender, for about 2 or 3 minutes.

CONCLUSION

Where does Dr. Sebi believe disease come from?

Doctor Sebi applied a bio-mineral, balanced approach to medicine rooted in African tradition. Instead of looking at diseases from germs, bacteria, or viruses, the disease is evaluated as developed where damage has been done to the mucus membrane, thereby compromising it.

By treating the patient with plant-based remedies, the body absorbs more alkaline substances, not 'harmful carcinogenic chemicals and poisons,' as Dr. Sebi describes. The disease can only exist in an acid environment. Specifically designed to replace lost or depleted minerals, his diet returns the body to an alkaline state while removing built-up toxins.

Doctor Sebi Diet seeks to support the primary organs responsible for eliminating body toxins. These organs that perform highly important body processing functions include:

Liver, Skin, Lymph glands, Kidneys, Gall bladder, and Colon.

Where the body cannot function as it should, these organs cannot effectively eliminate toxins. This inability to flush out itself results in an accumulation of toxins in the body that end up being recycled in the body, eventually manifesting disease.

The shocking truth Dr. Sebi teaches is that the body begins to malfunction in this toxic state and effectively break down weaker organs due to its inability to purge these harmful toxins.

Doctor Sebi's methodology identifies the colon as the most important organ of all listed organs. Sebi teaches to be cleaned and detoxified before successful steps can be taken to treat and reverse the effects of the disease.

As important as colon cleaning in Doctor Sebi Diet, the focus of the diet is ultimately holistic. If your colon is the single organ that is detoxified and cleaned, all other non-detoxified and cleaned organs will still retain toxicity, resulting in the body remaining in a diseased state.

Dorothy Vandekamp.

Printed in Great Britain
by Amazon